Diane Fisher

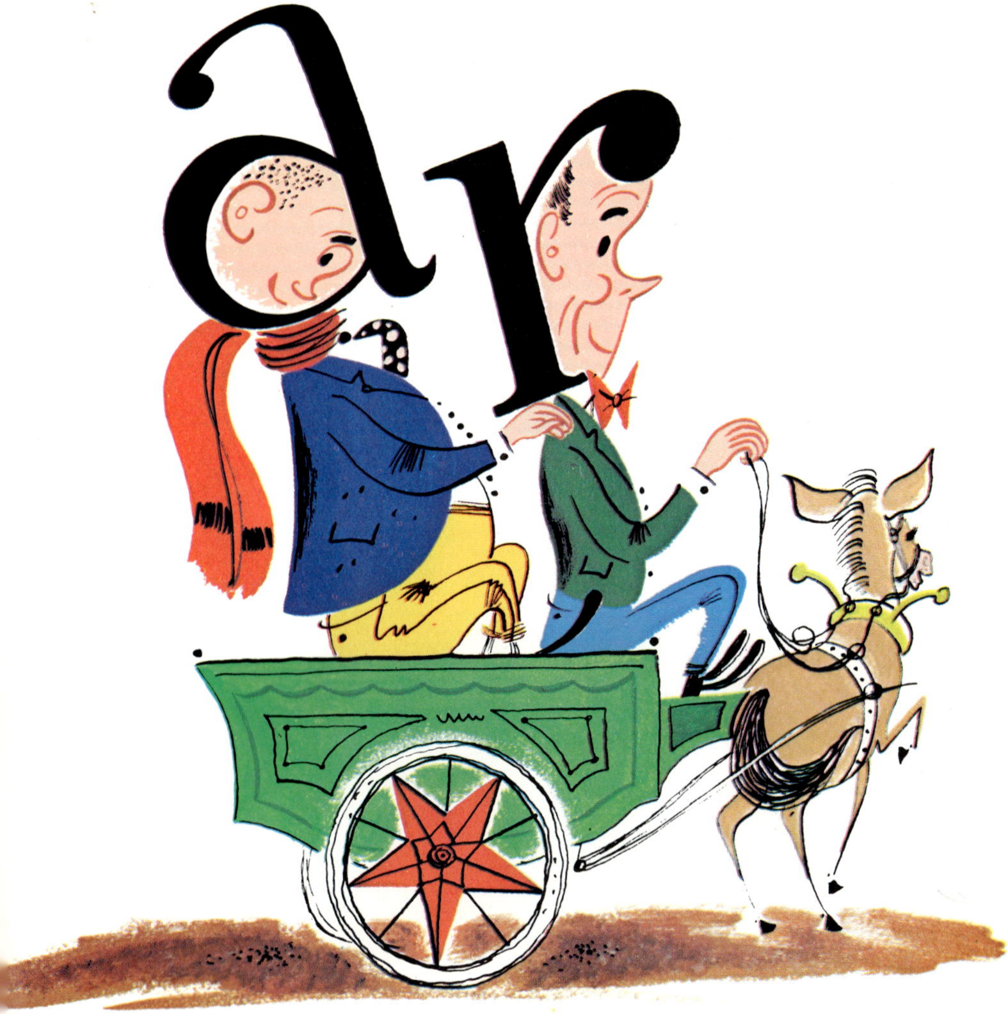

ar

arm darn tar dart tart cart

art card mar hard harm part

star car farm far scarf

are

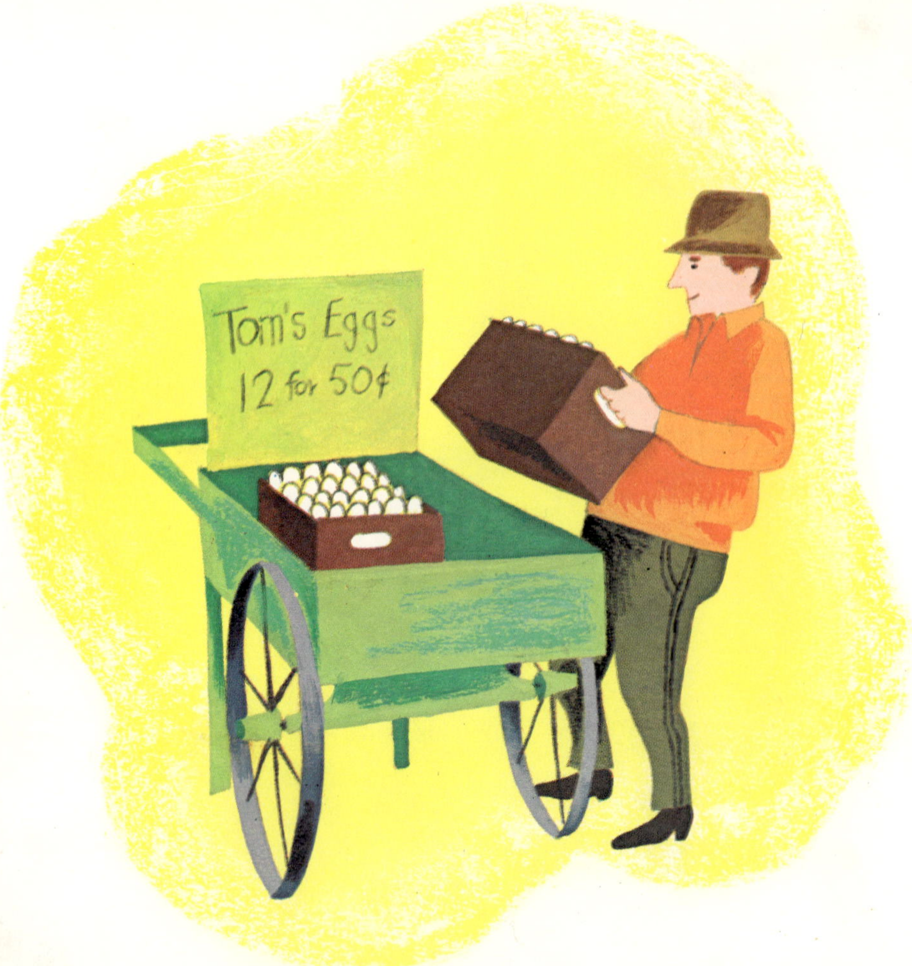

The Cats and the Cart

Tom is a farm hand.
Tom has a farm cart.

A card is on the cart.
Tom puts eggs in his cart.

puts

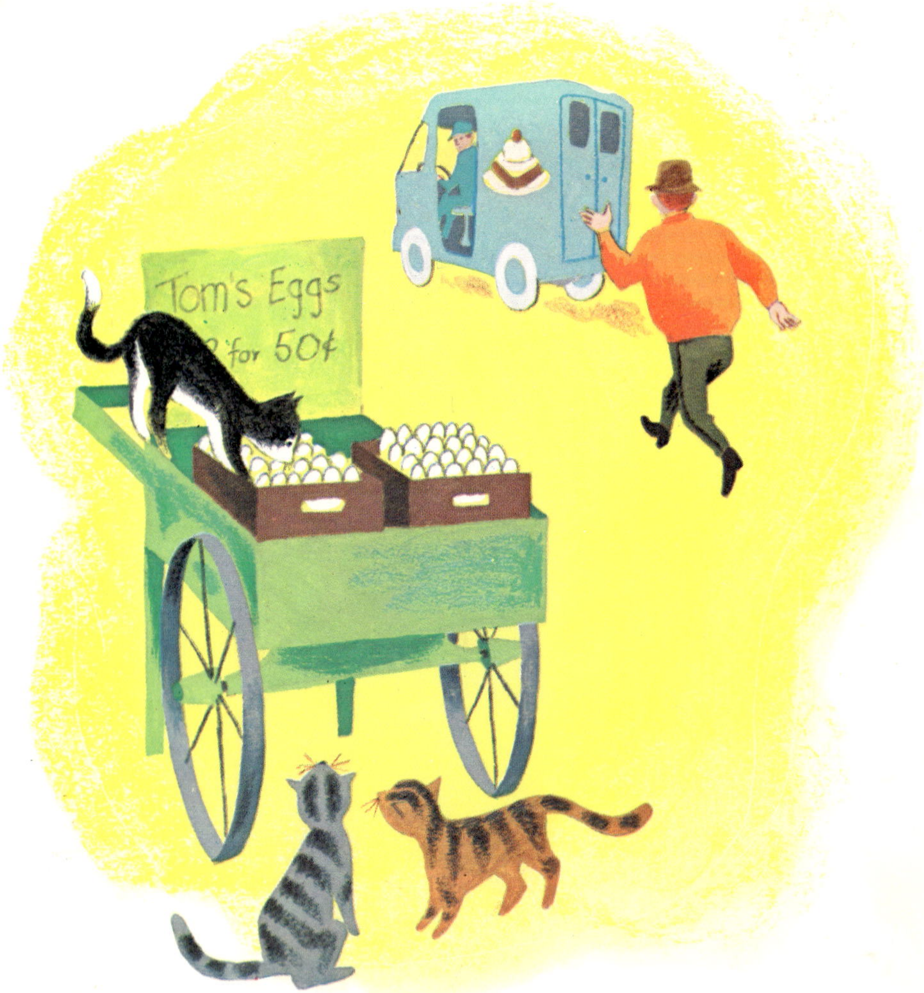

Tom runs off to get a tart.
Tom is far from the cart.

The cats are at the cart.

to

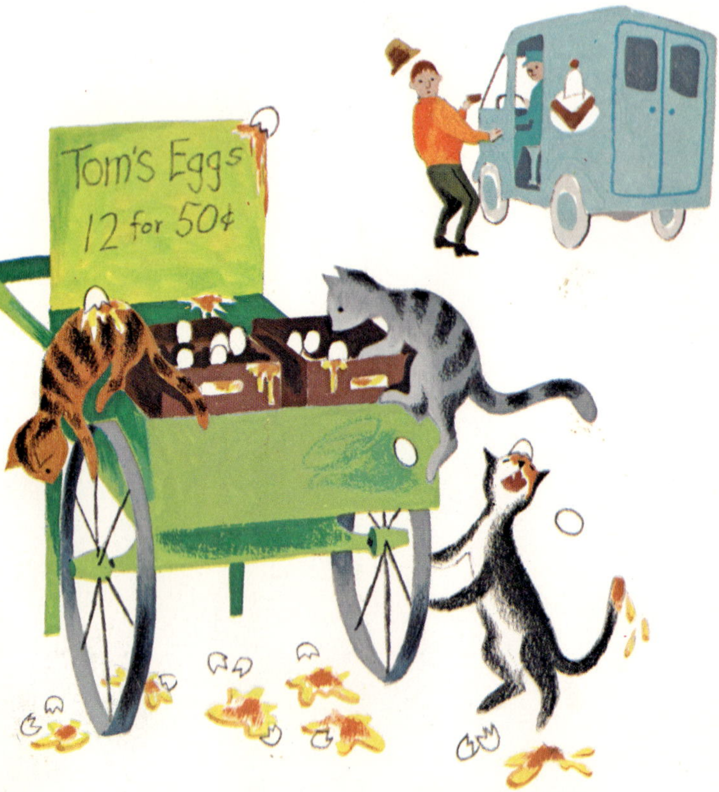

Can the cats harm the eggs?
The cats harm the eggs.
And the eggs harm the cats.

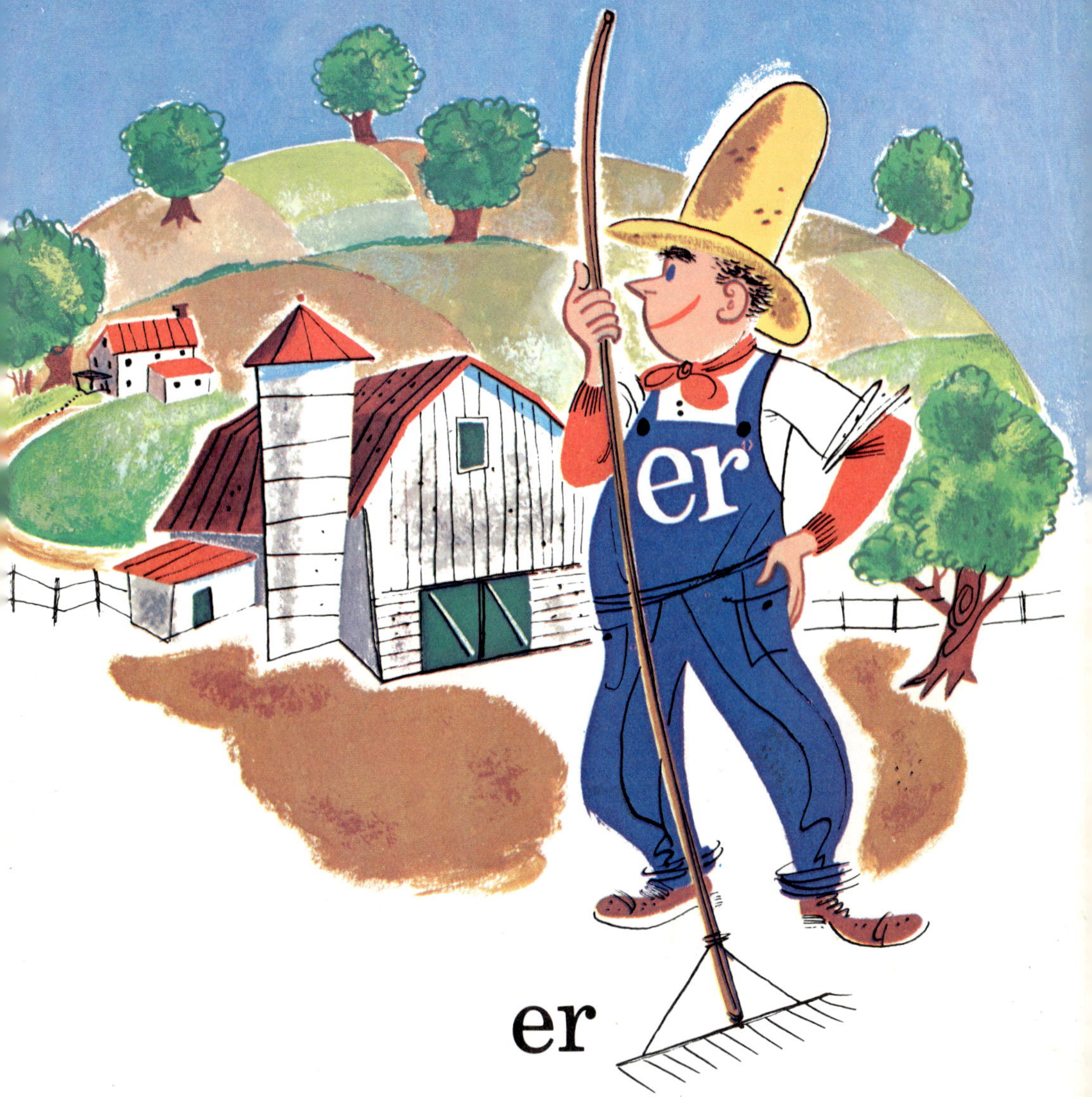

er

fast	faster	start	starter
tend	tender	hunt	hunter
wet	wetter	camp	camper
farm	farmer	mend	mender
her			

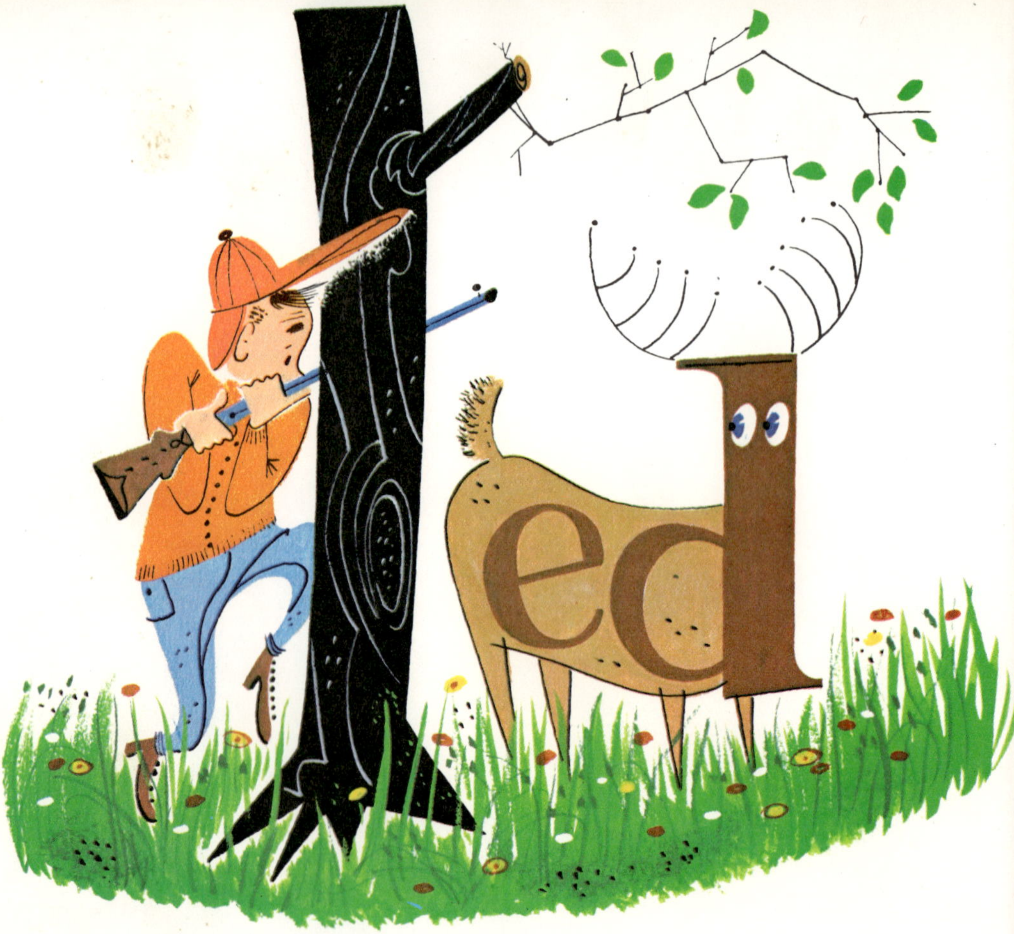

ed

hand	handed	mend	mended
start	started	hunt	hunted
dent	dented	dart	darted

into upon after across under garden

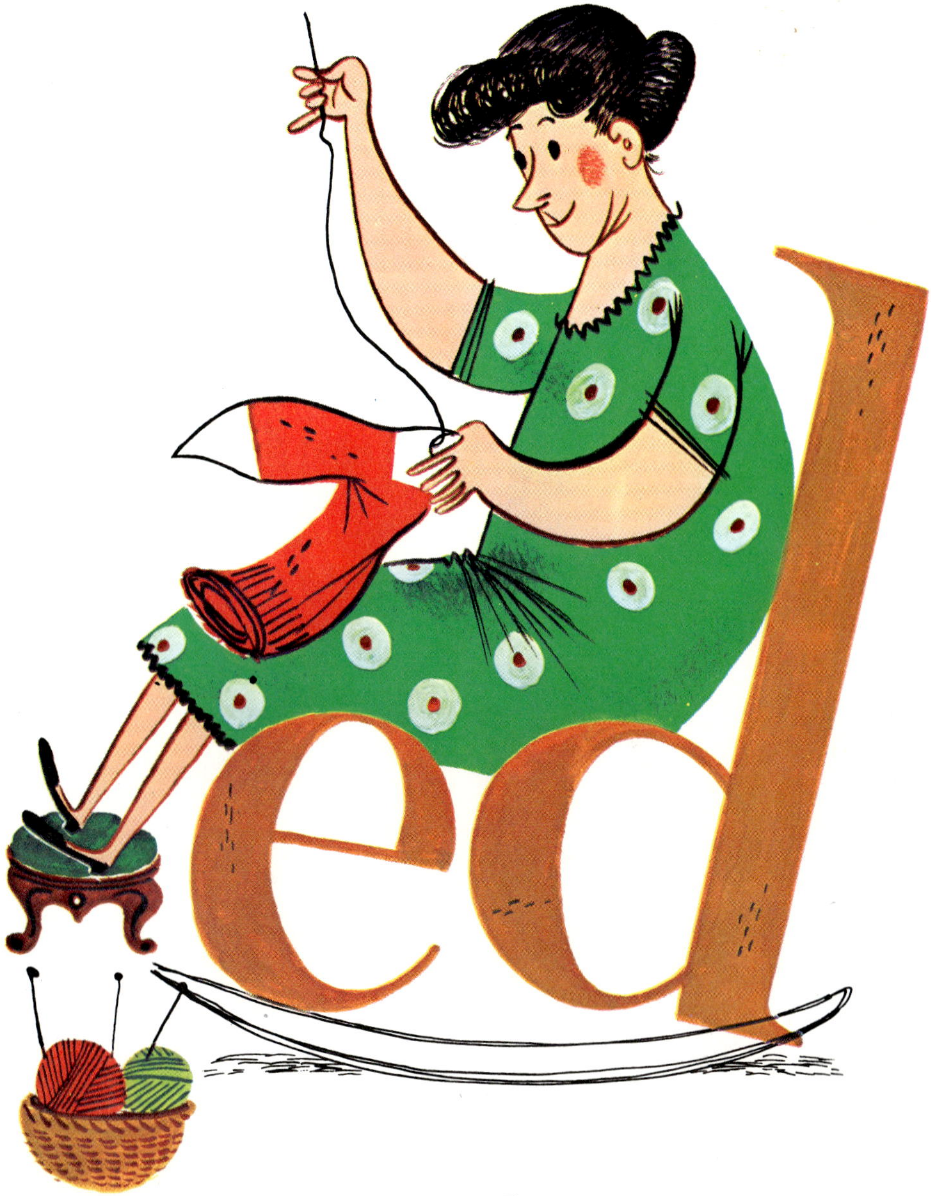

ed

farm farmed

harm harmed darn darned

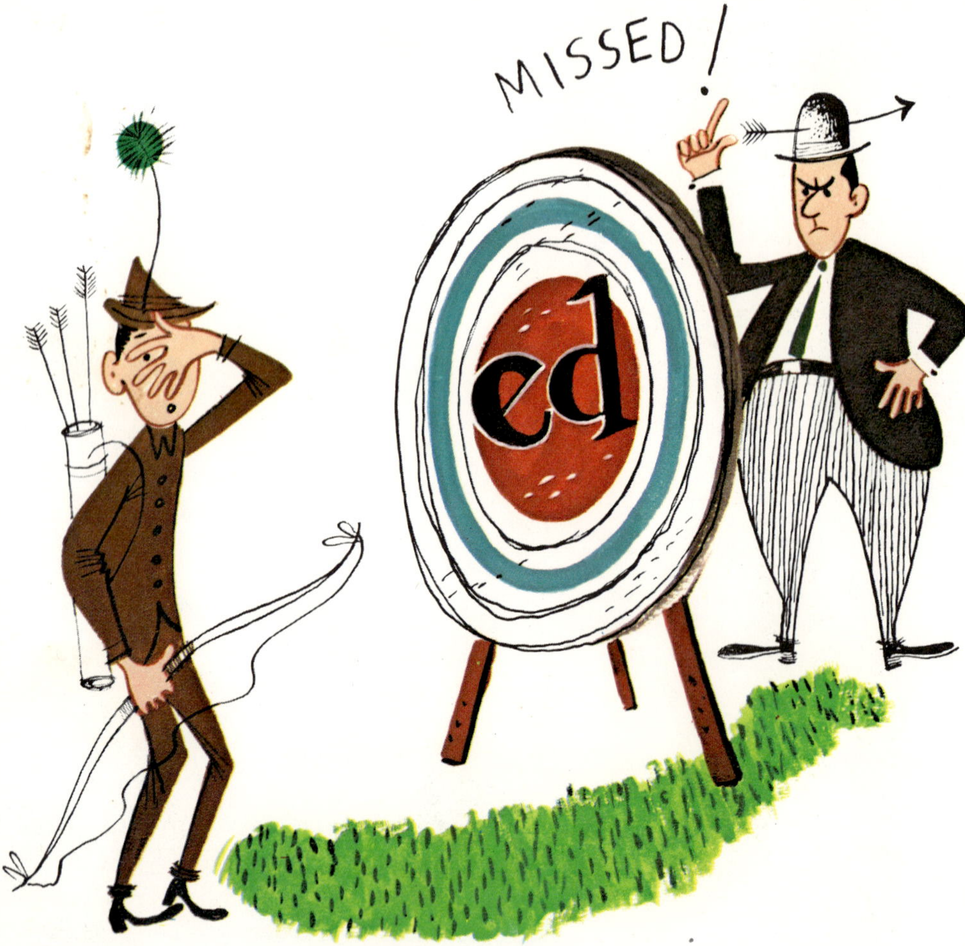

ed

camp	camped	stop	stopped
cross	crossed	snap	snapped
stamp	stamped	miss	missed
gasp	gasped	toss	tossed

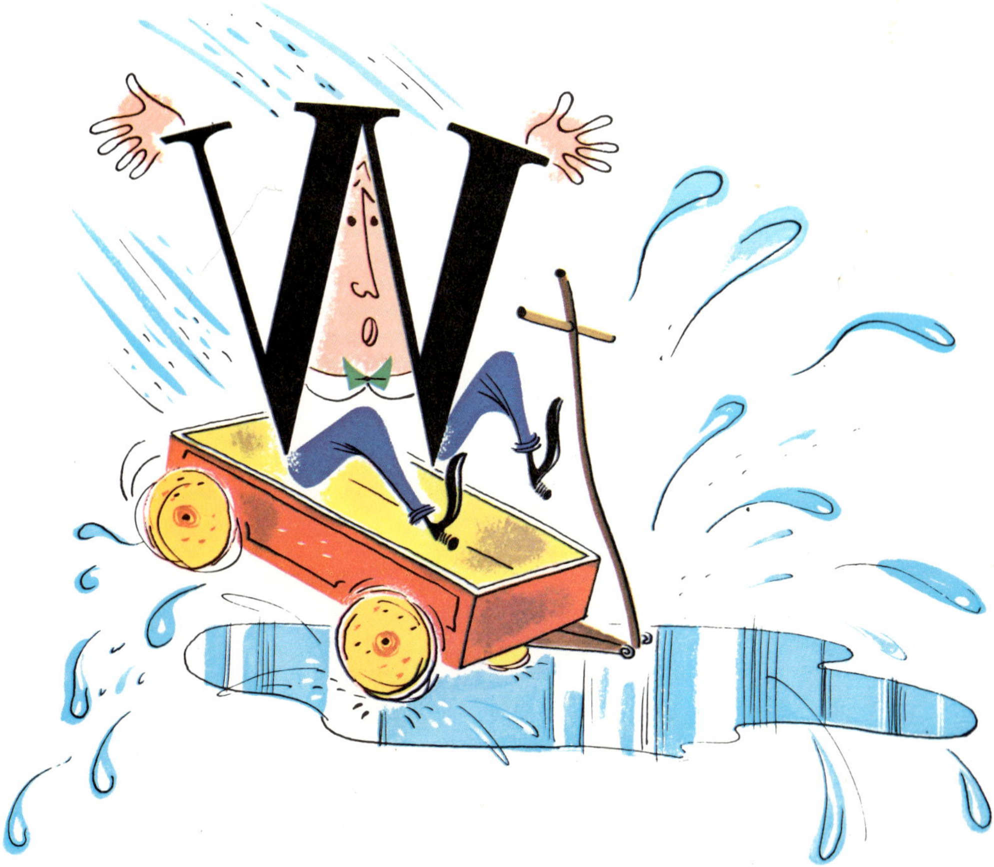

w W

wet went wig wag win
winter west western wagon

water want wasp was

were

Wags Gets Wet

Wags, the dog, got into the wagon.
It was a red wagon.

The wagon started to run fast.
Faster and faster it went.

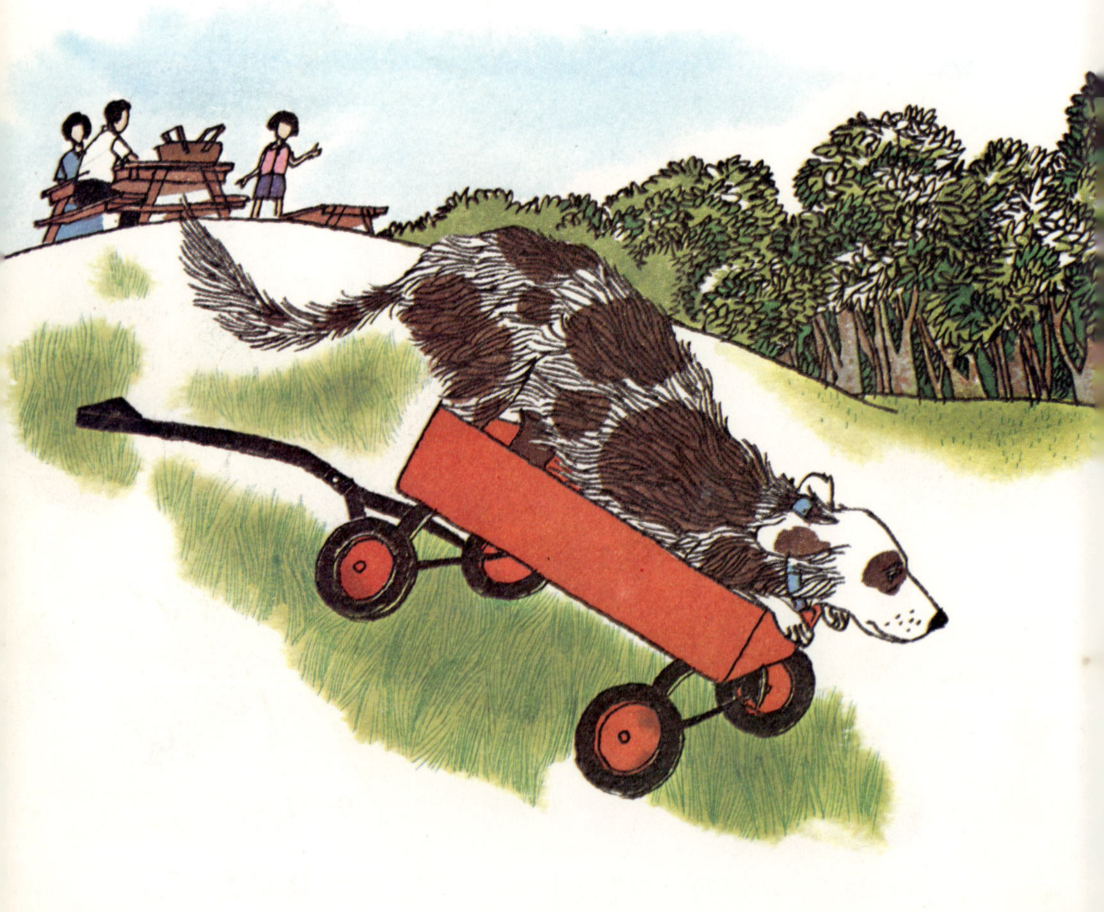

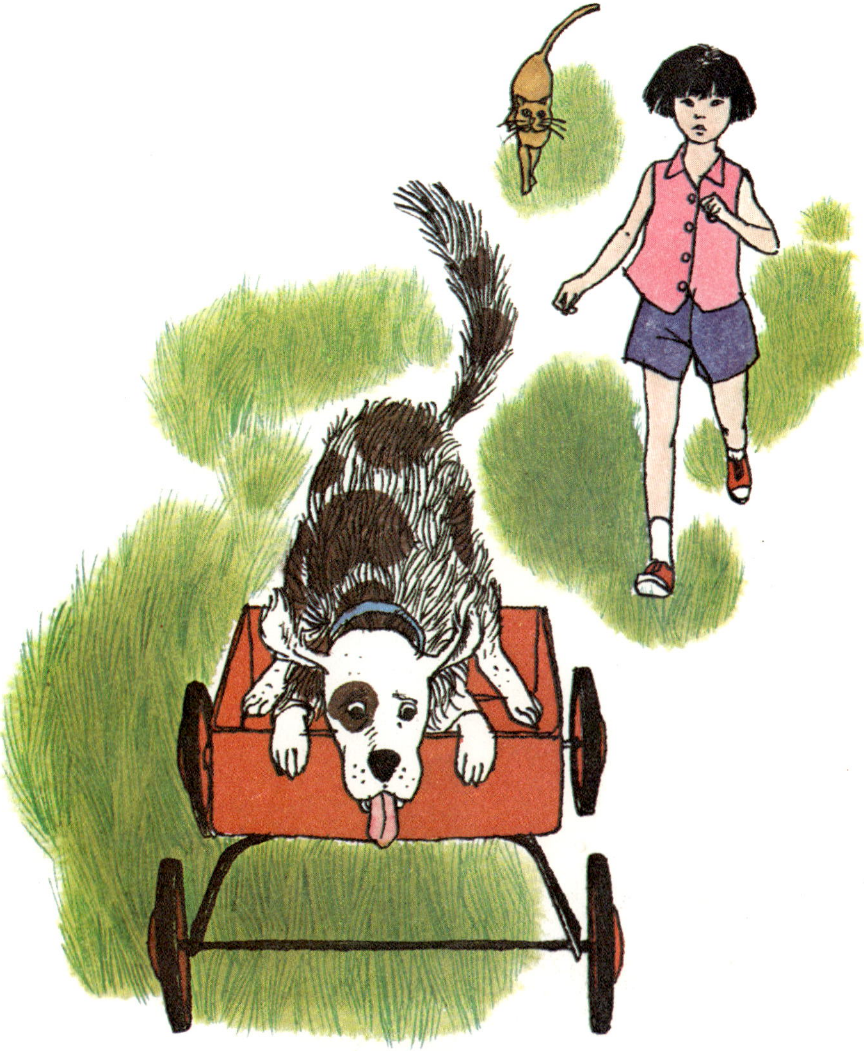

Pam darted after it.
Topper, the cat, ran after Pam.

Pam wanted to stop the wagon.
Wags must not get harmed.

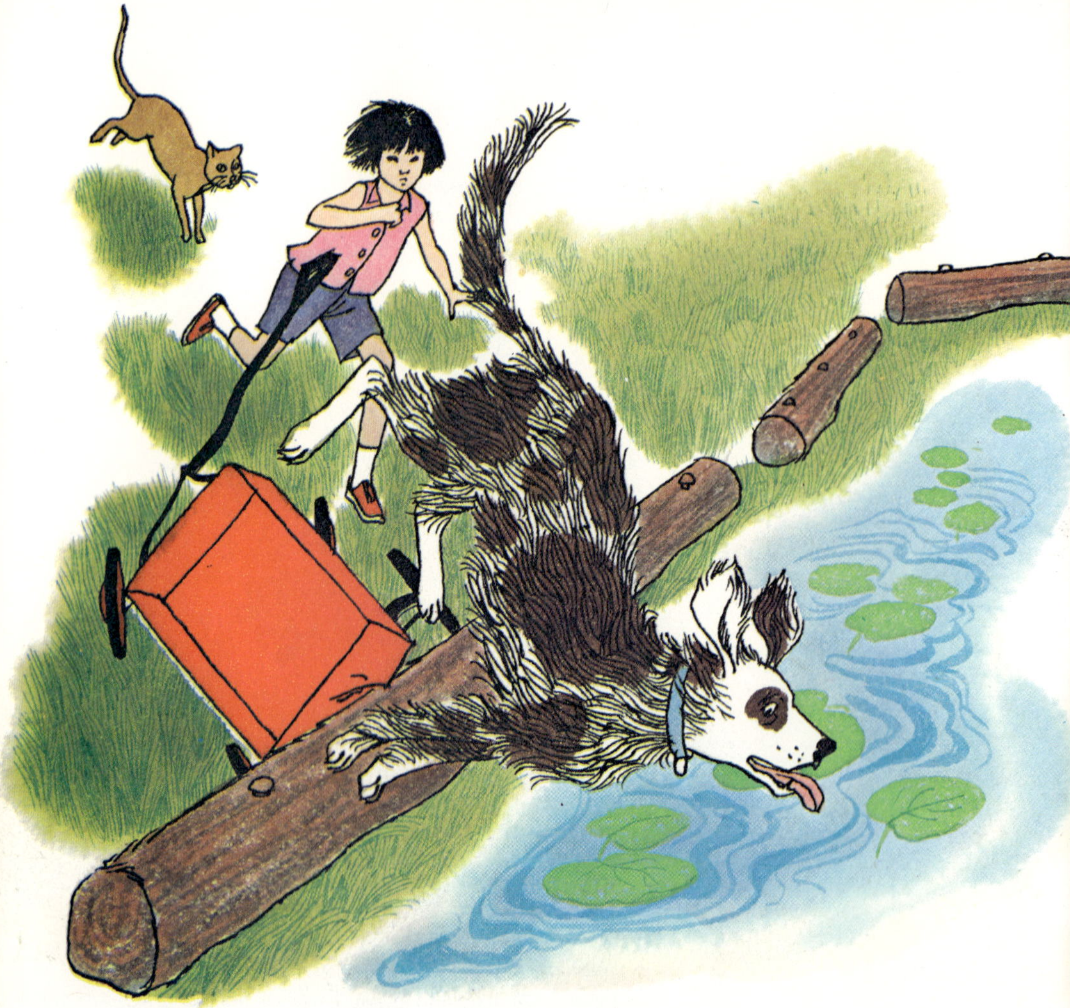

The wagon stopped at the pond.
Wags did not stop.

Into the water went Wags!
Pam darted in after him.

Pam and Wags got wet.
Wags was not harmed.

The red wagon hit hard.
It was dented.

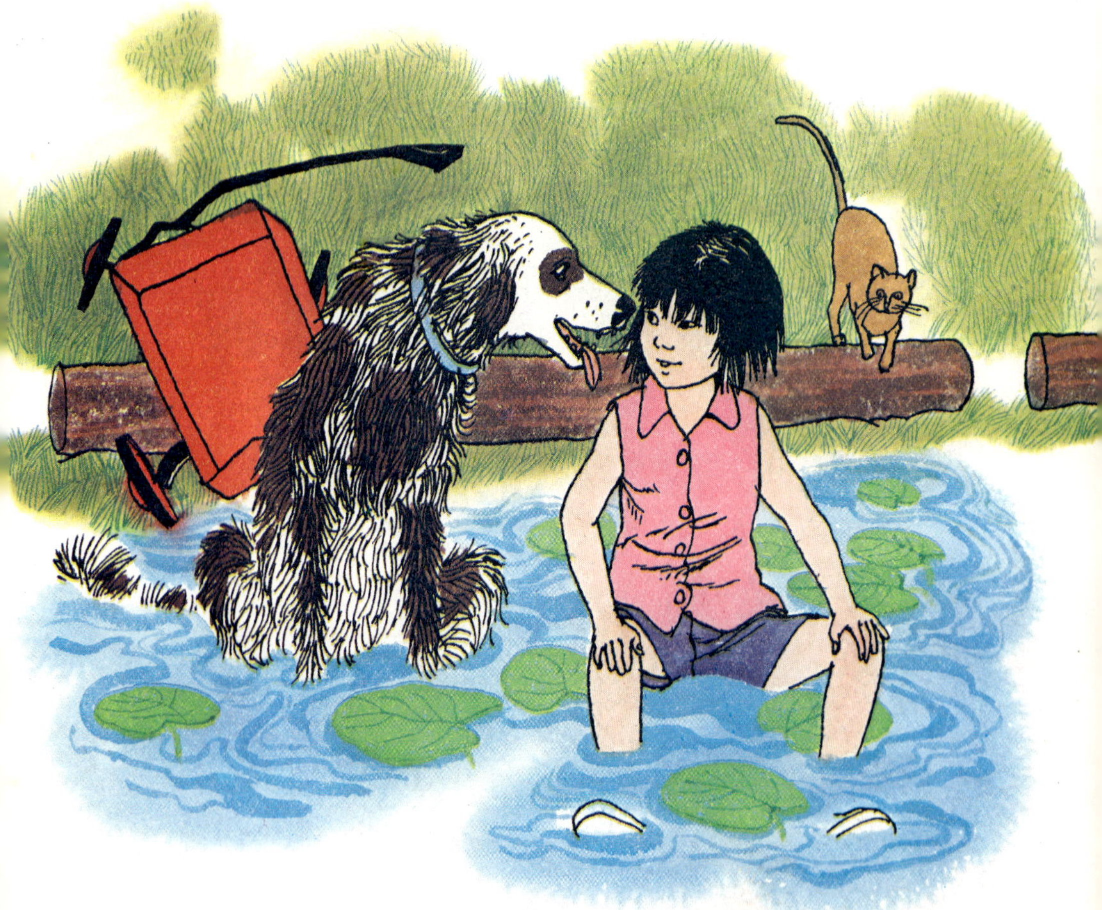

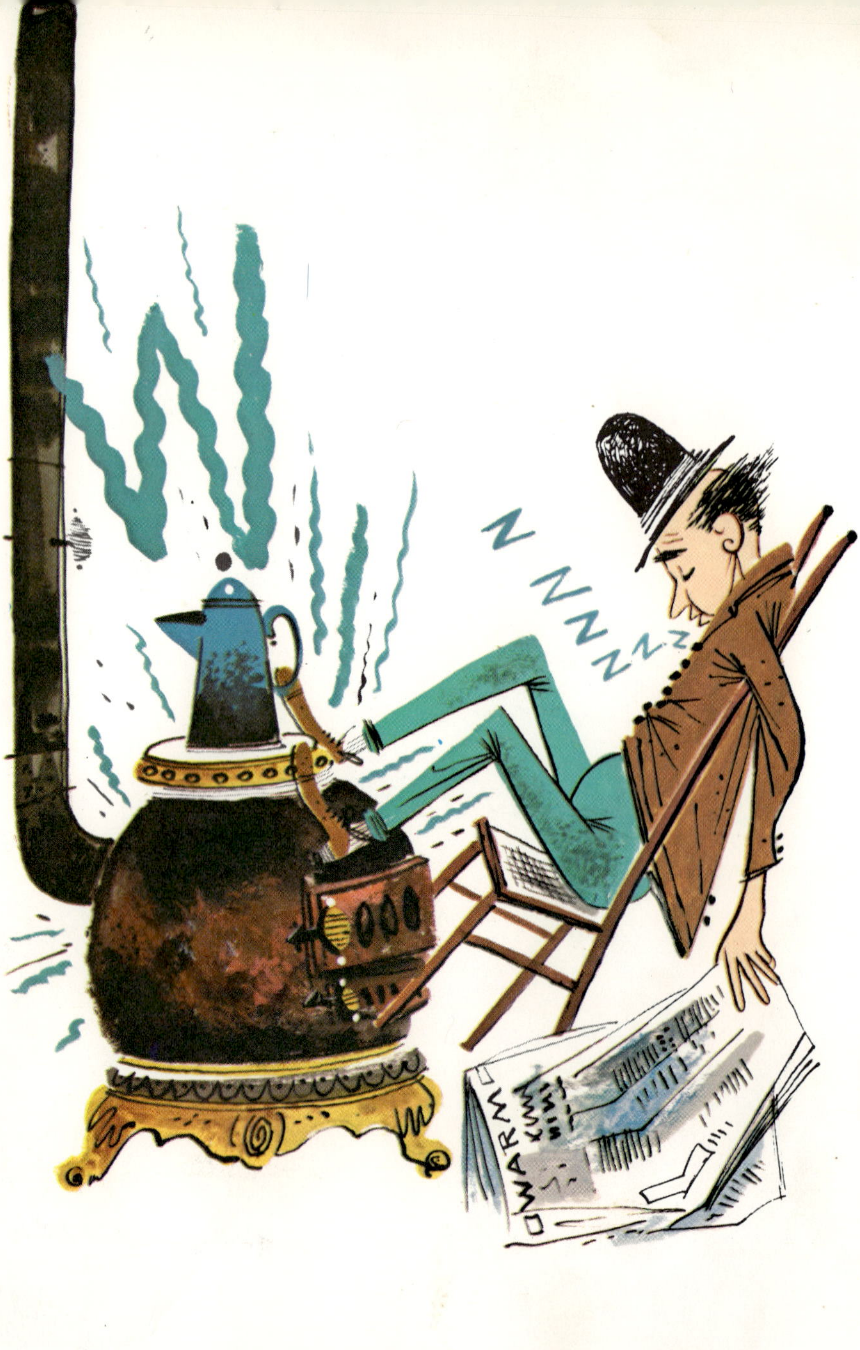

w W

war wart warm swarm

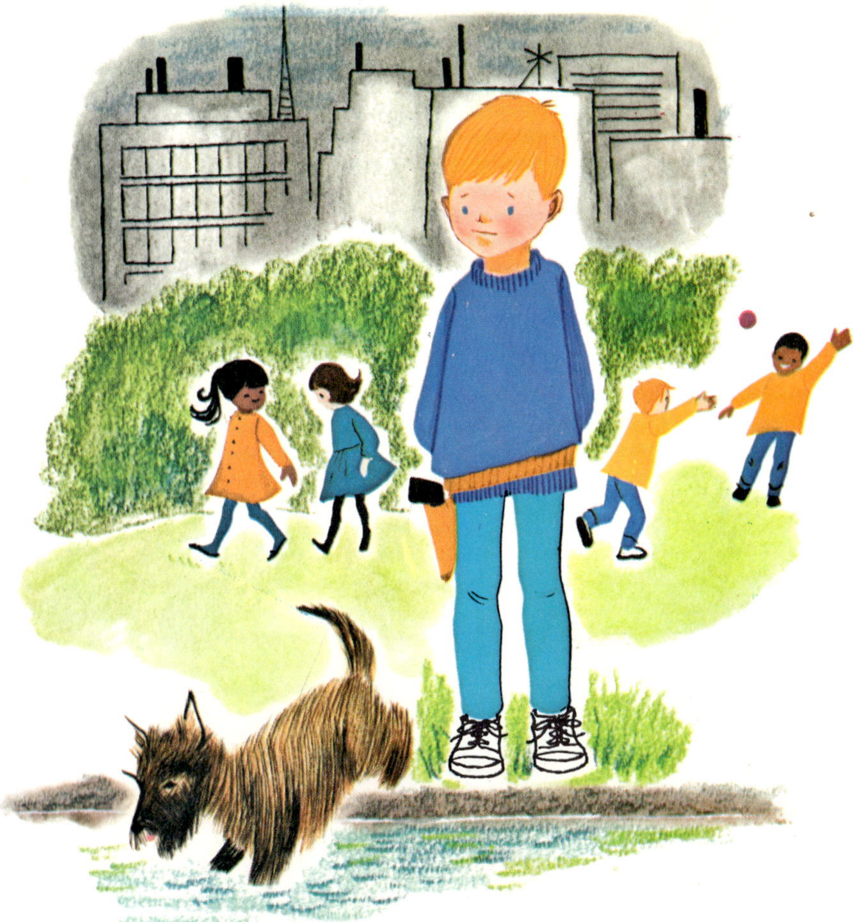

Ted and Rags

Rags ran into the water.
The water was warm.

Ted wanted to run in the water.
Ted did not want to get wet.
Rags got wetter and wetter.

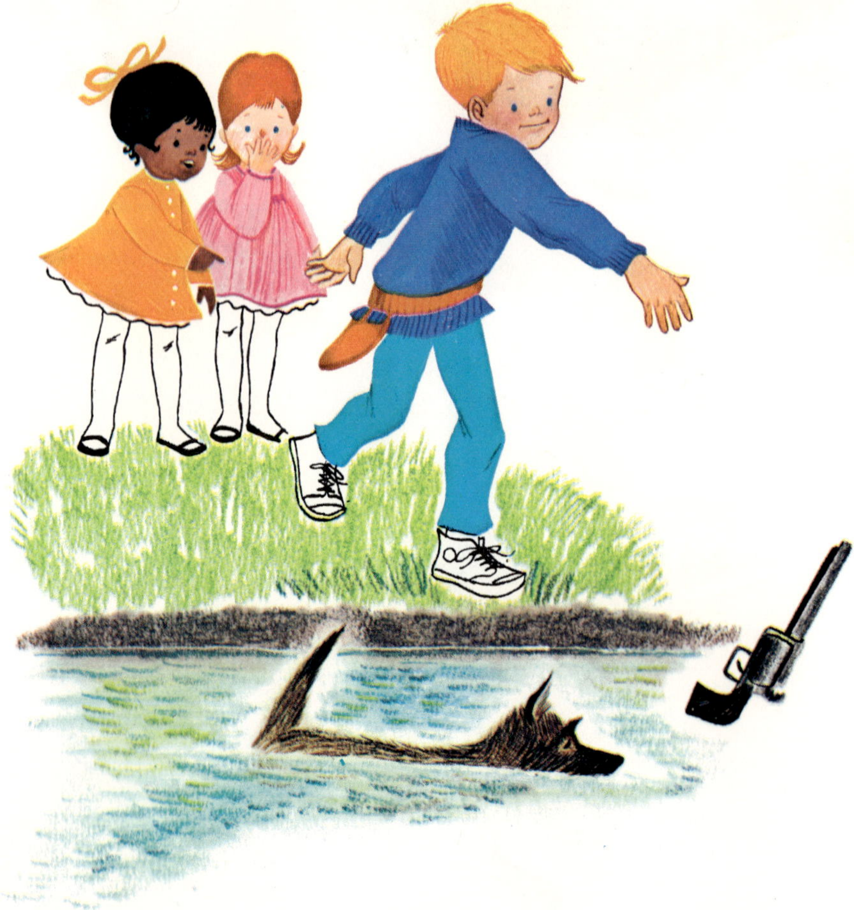

“Get it, Rags, get it,” said Ted.
“Get the gun in the water.”

Rags went to get the gun.
Rags got wetter and wetter.

said

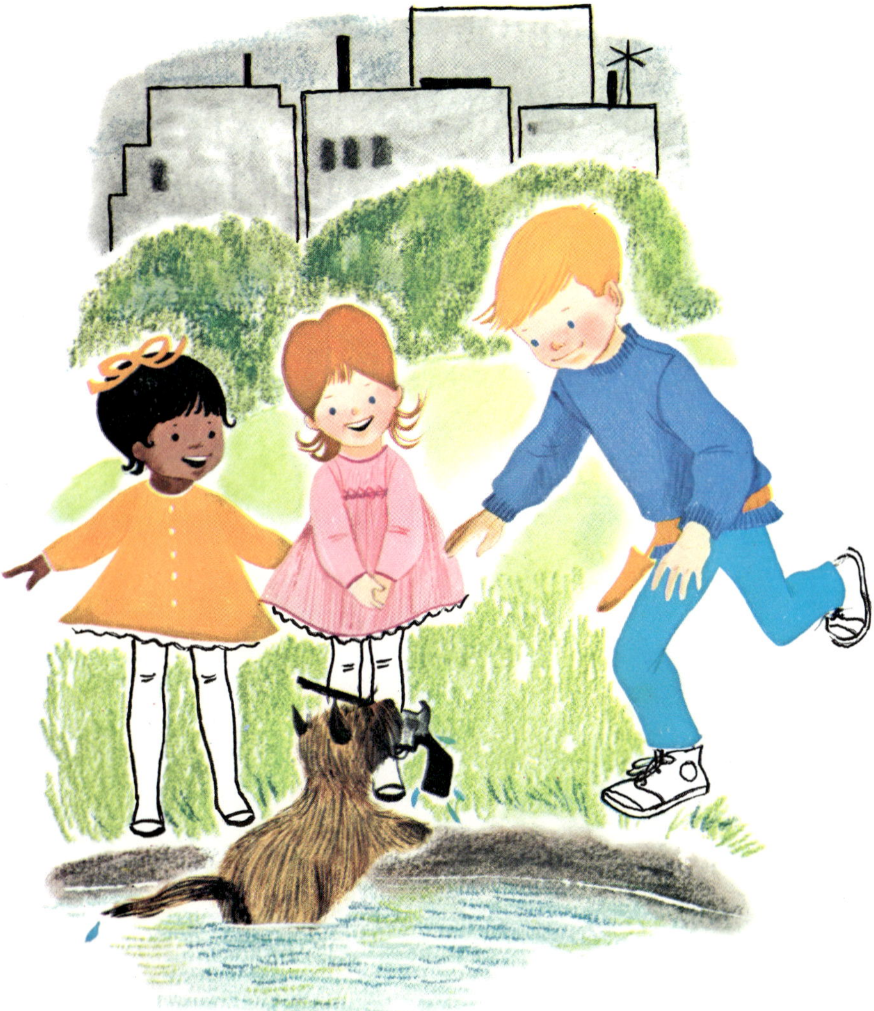

Rags got the gun for Ted.
Ted went to Rags to get it.

Rags was wet.
Rags got the water off.

for

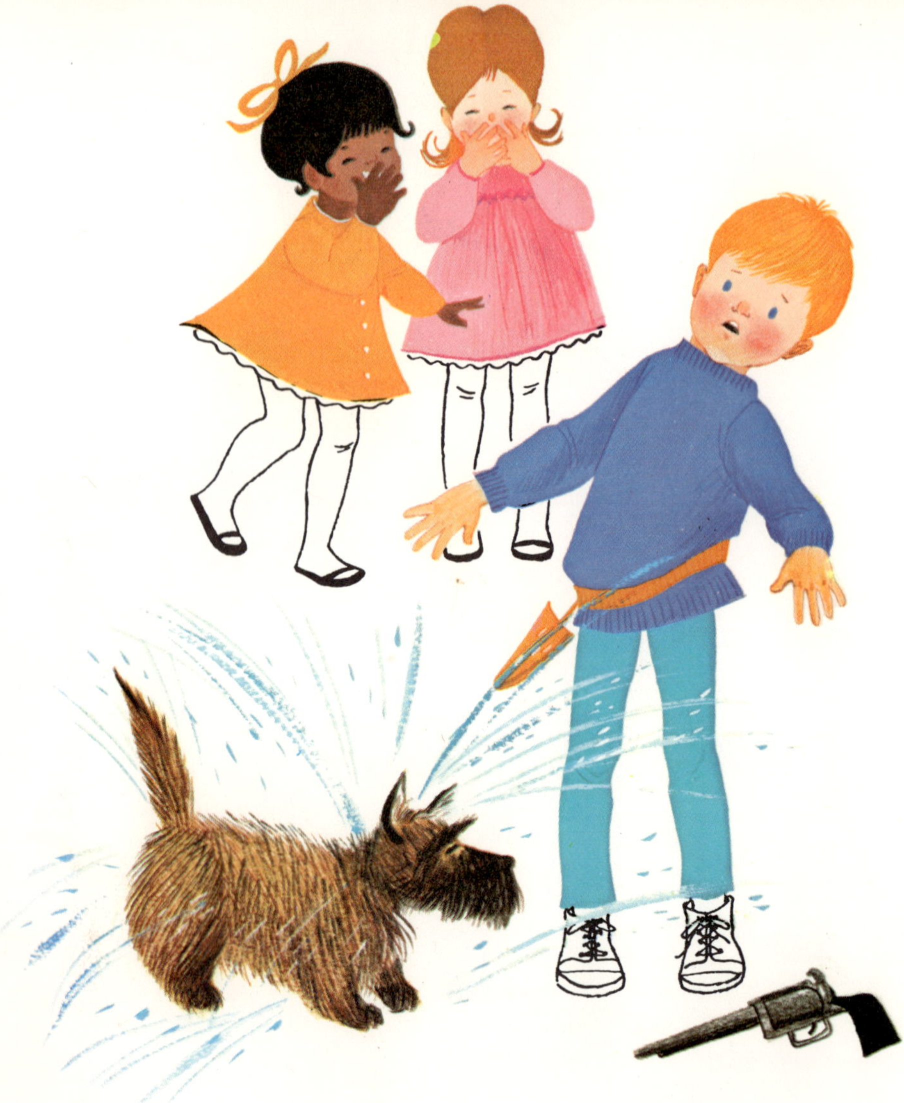

The water went from him to Ted.
The water was on Ted.

"The water is wet," said Ted.
"The water is wet and warm."

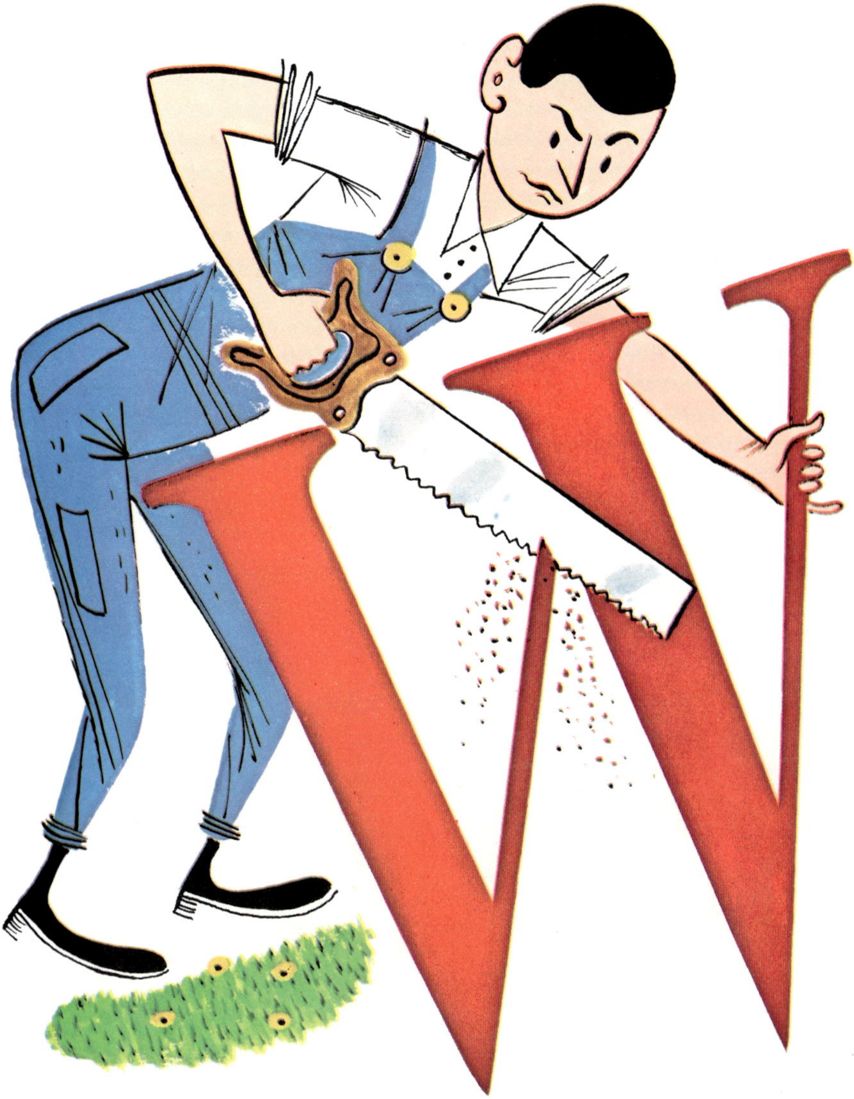

aw

saw paw raw caw

draw dawn fawn

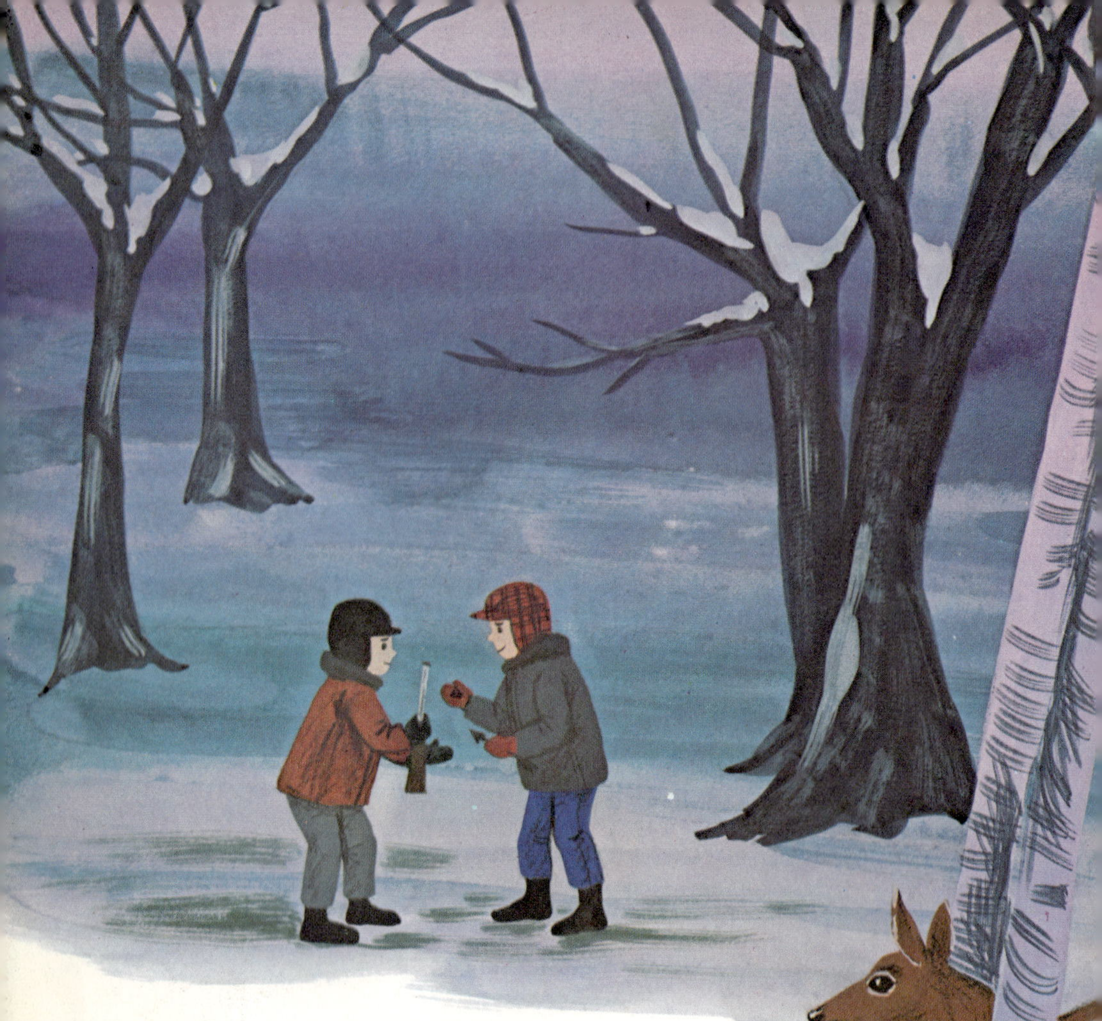

A Fawn at Dawn

Sam handed Win a gun.
Win handed Sam a dart.

Sam and Win went into the forest.
Fawns were in the forest.

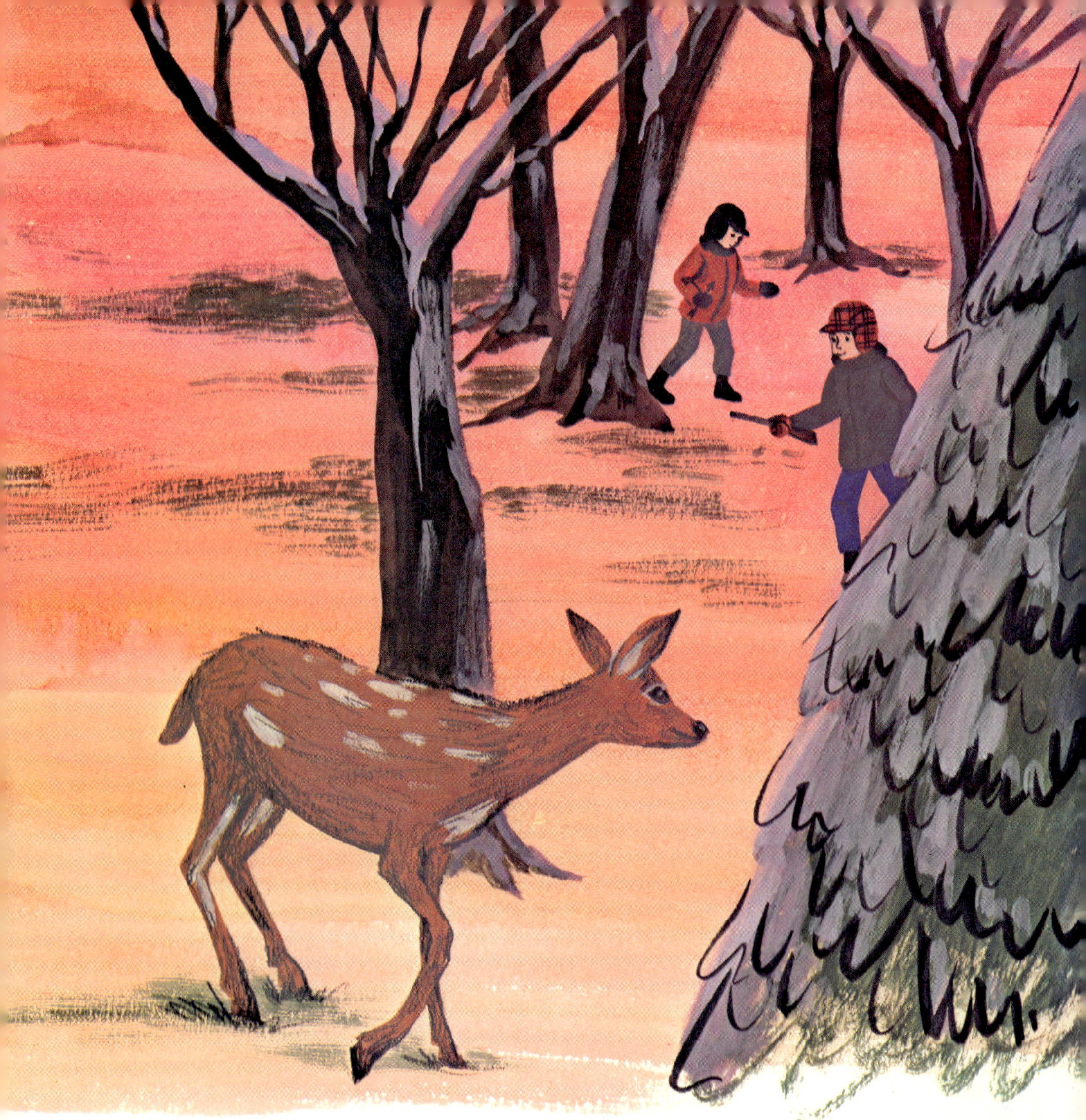

At dawn, Win saw a fat fawn.
The fawn saw Sam and Win.

It started to run fast.
It ran into a winter camp tent.

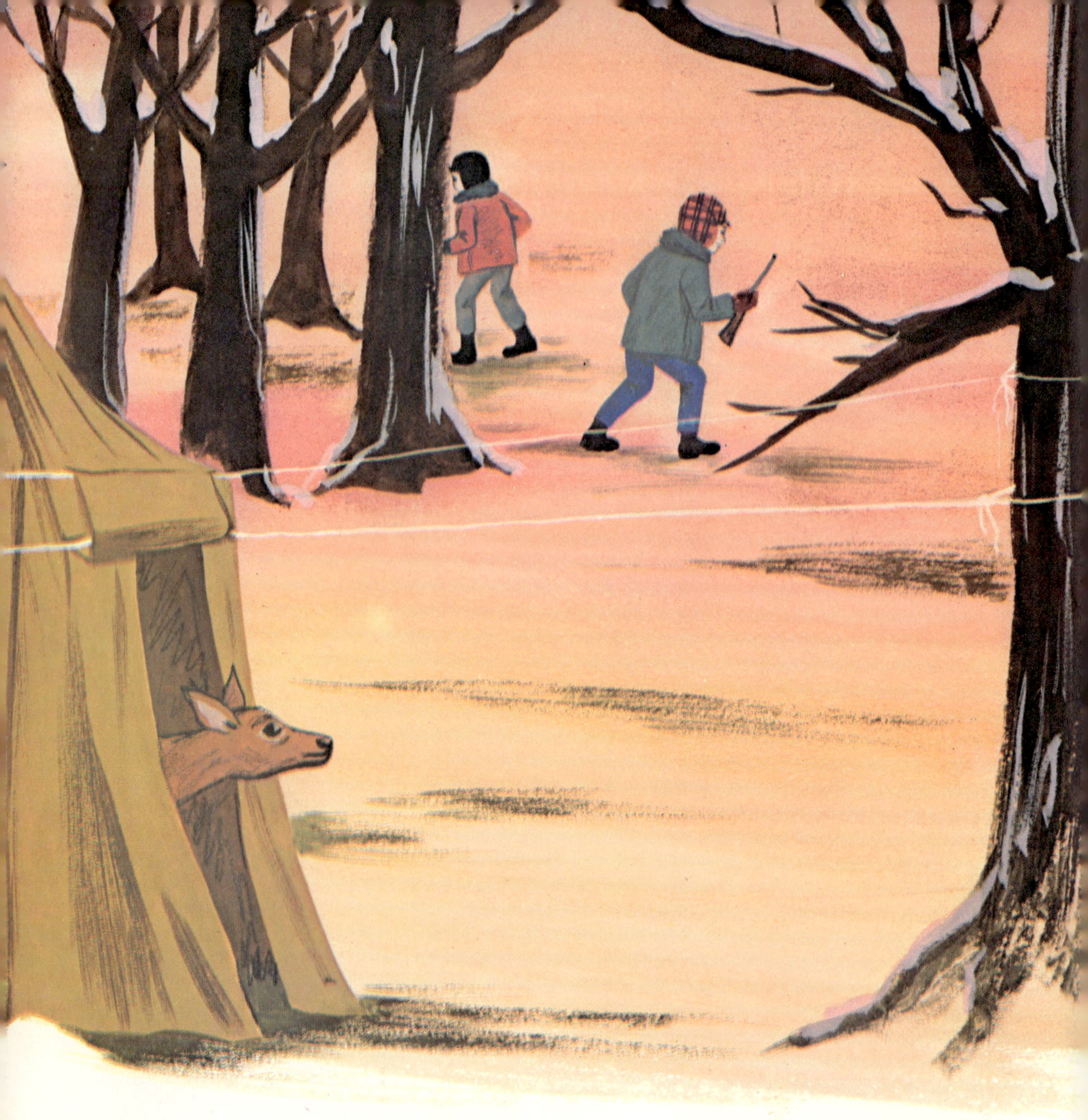

Sam and Win hunted for the fawn.
It hid in the tent.

Sam started to the farm.
Sam must not harm a fawn.

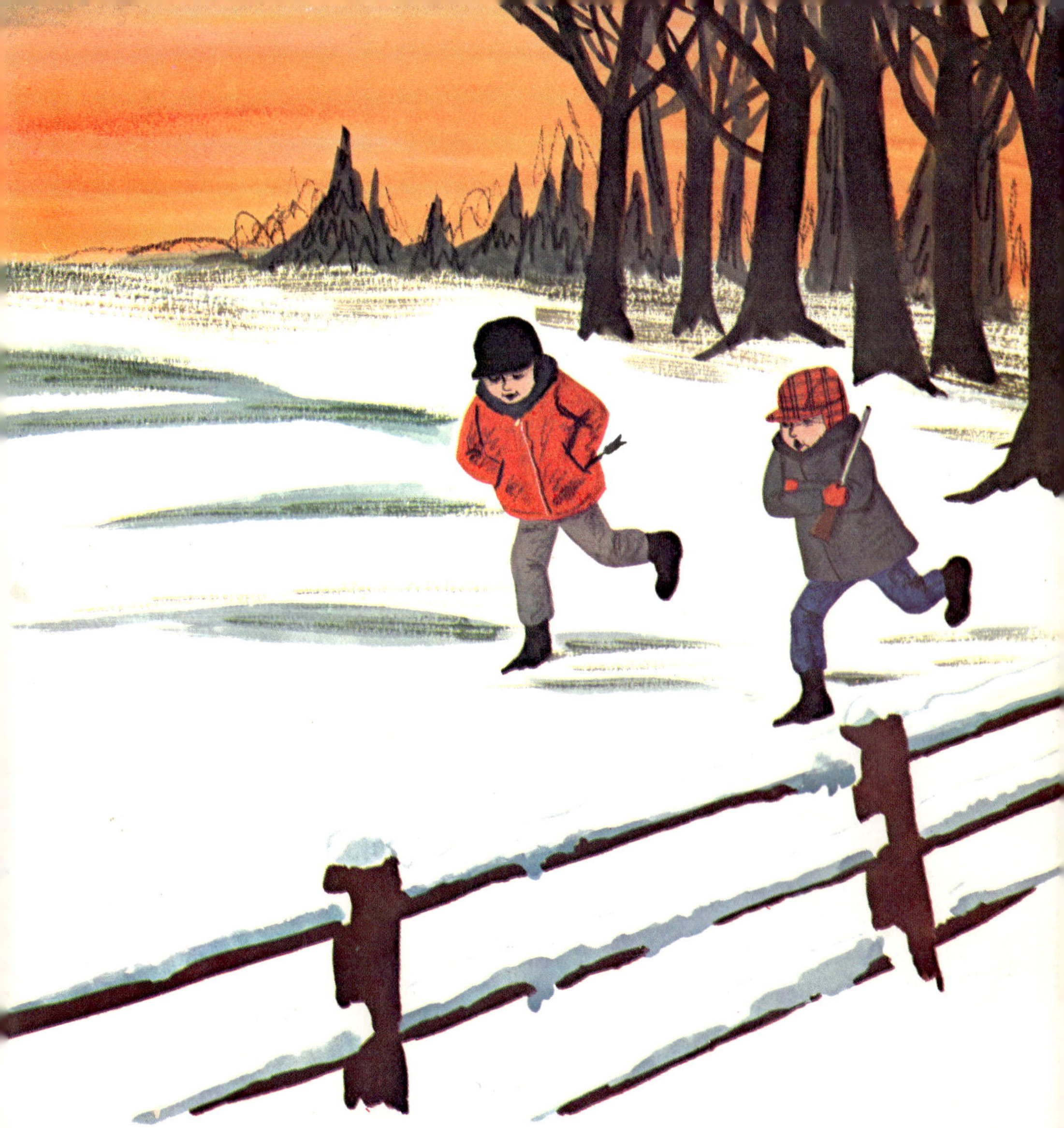

Win and Sam went to the farm.
Win wanted to get warm.

The raw winter dug into his hands.
Win and Sam did not harm the fawn.

ow

how now cow down town

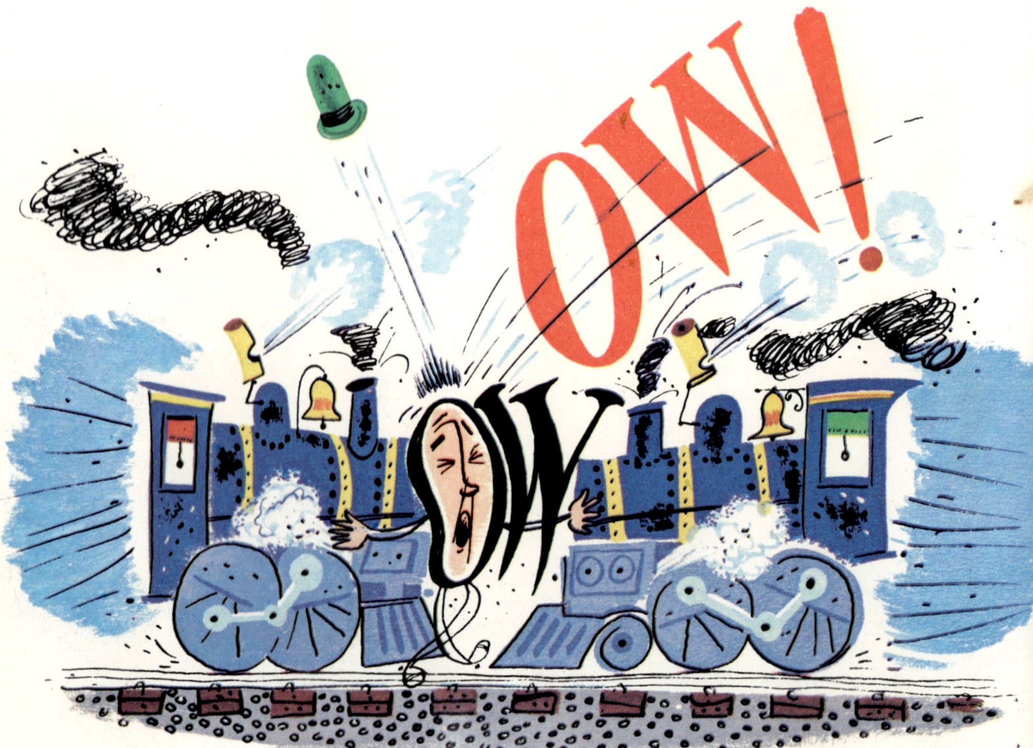

The Cow and the Frog

A fat frog sat on a raft.

A tan cow saw the fat frog.

The cow sat down on the raft.

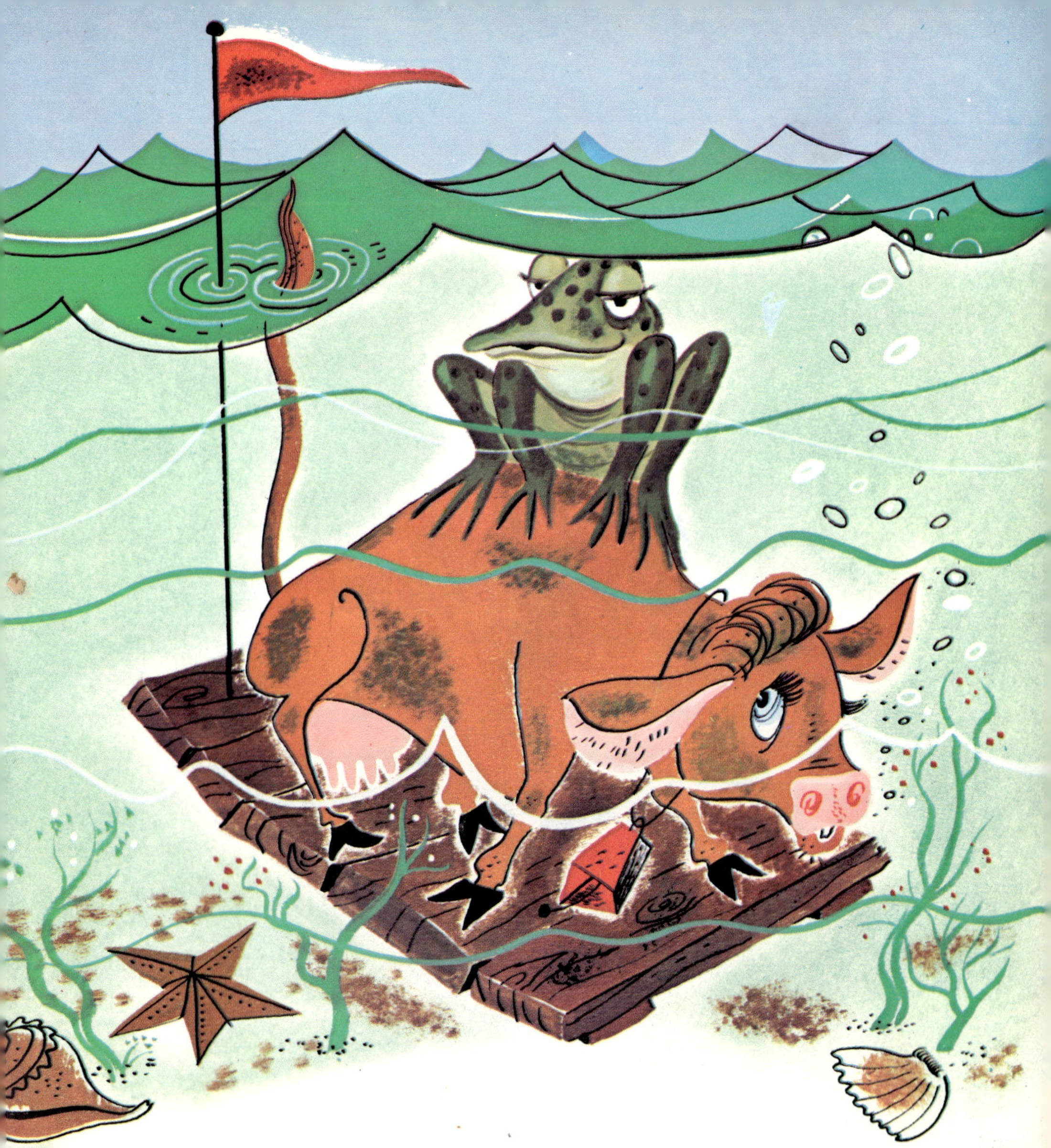

Down, down went the raft.
It went down into the water.

Now the cow sits in the water.
The frog sits on the cow.

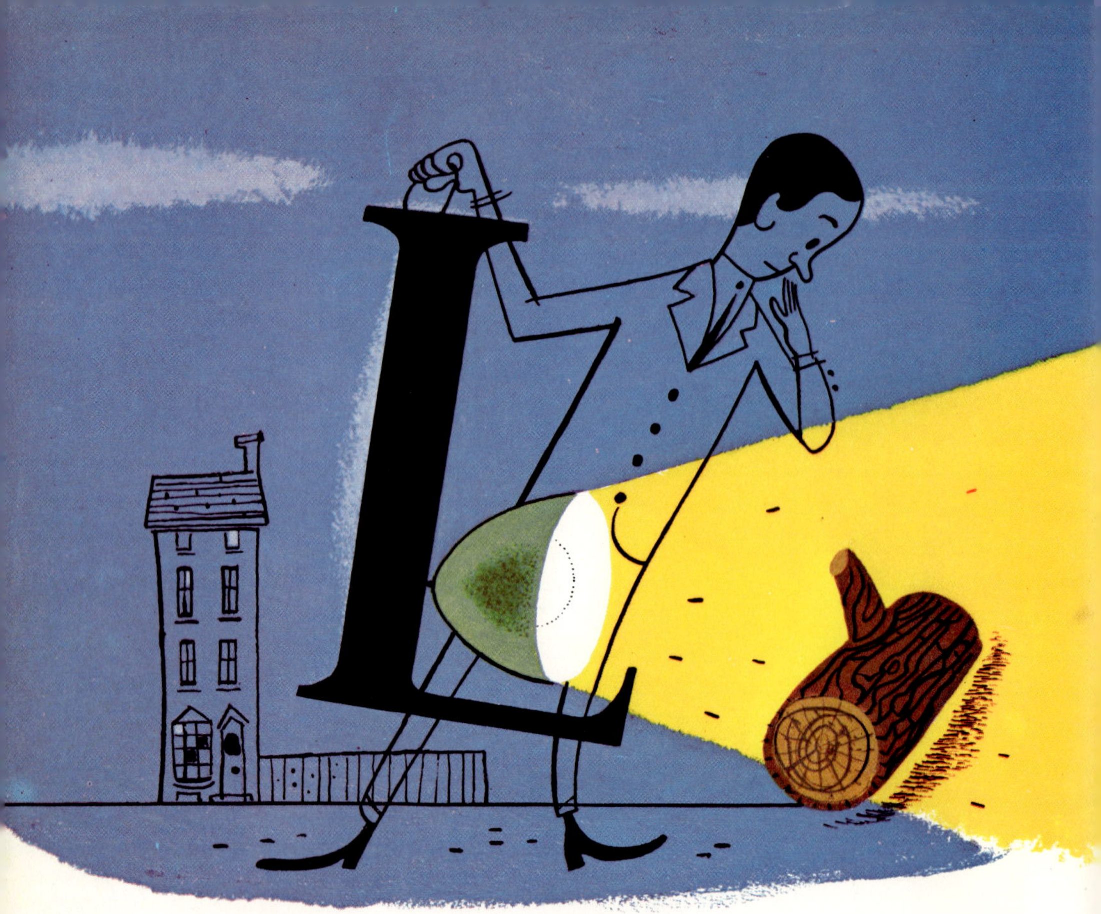

l L

lot	lad	log	lap	let	letter
lip	last	less	lamp	list	lost

clan	class	clap	clod	clam	slip
sled	slap	slit	slop	slam	glad
flat	flag	flip	flop	plot	plug
plan	plant	held	help	helmet	antler

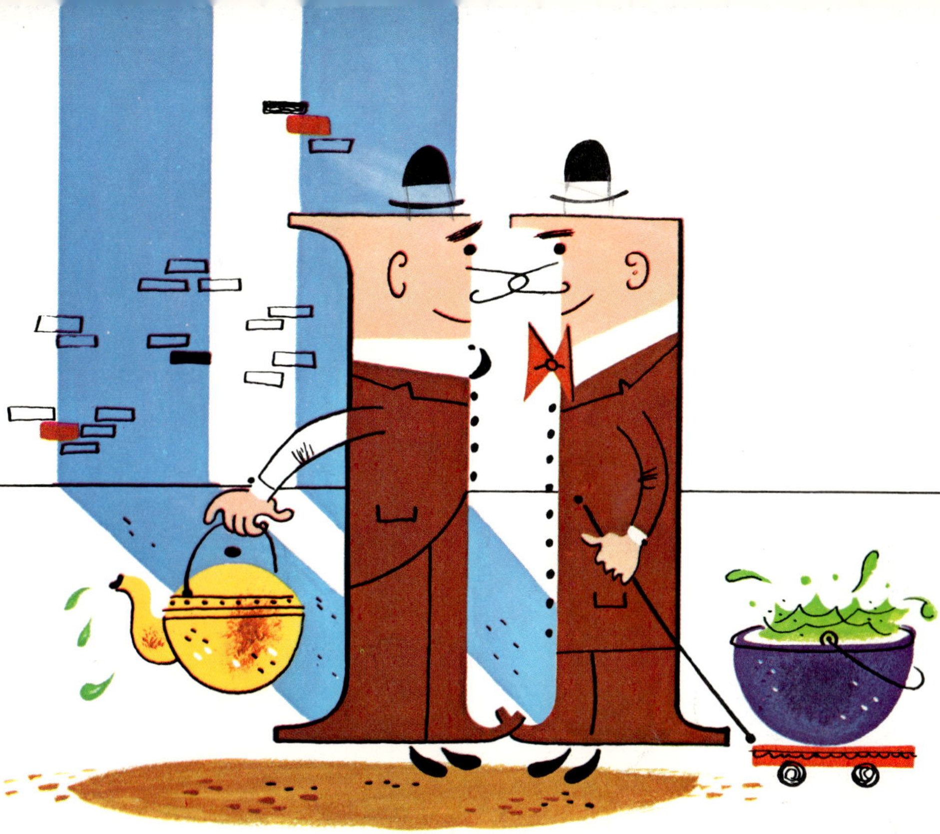

ll

all	tall	fall	call	hall	stall
wall	fell	well	will	hill	till
mill	pill	sill	small	still	

pull full pullet

Pull the full pan.

Put the water in the pot.

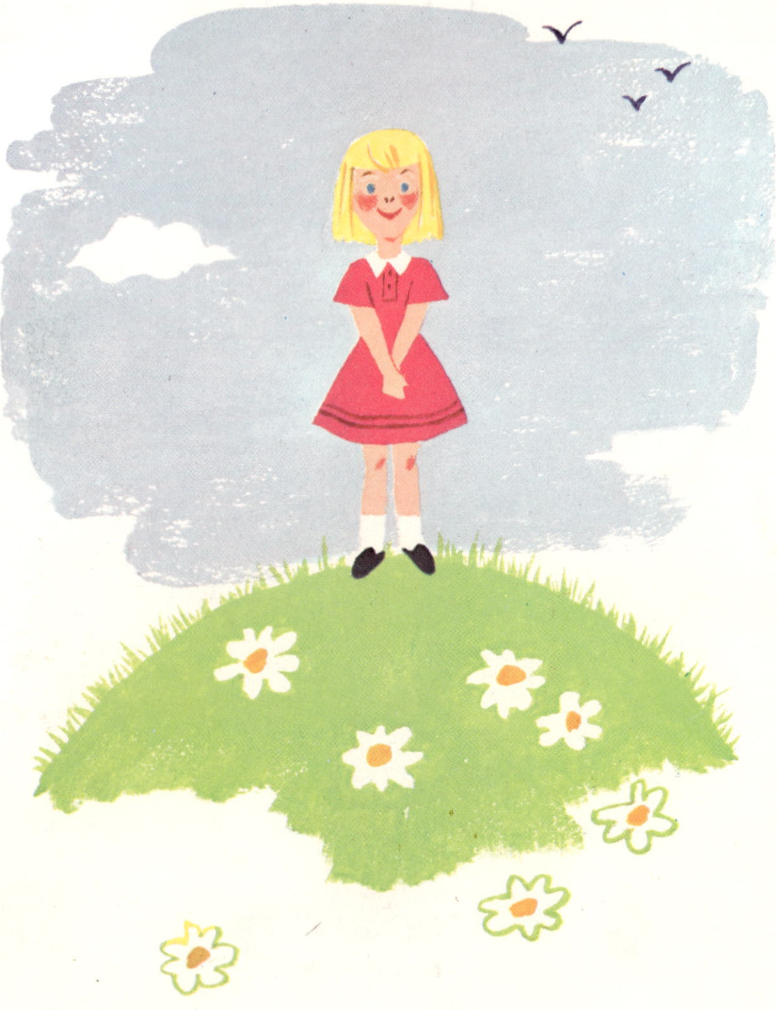

Ellen on a hill-top
Ellen on a hill
Ellen on a hill-top-hill
Still, still, still

Adele H. Seronde

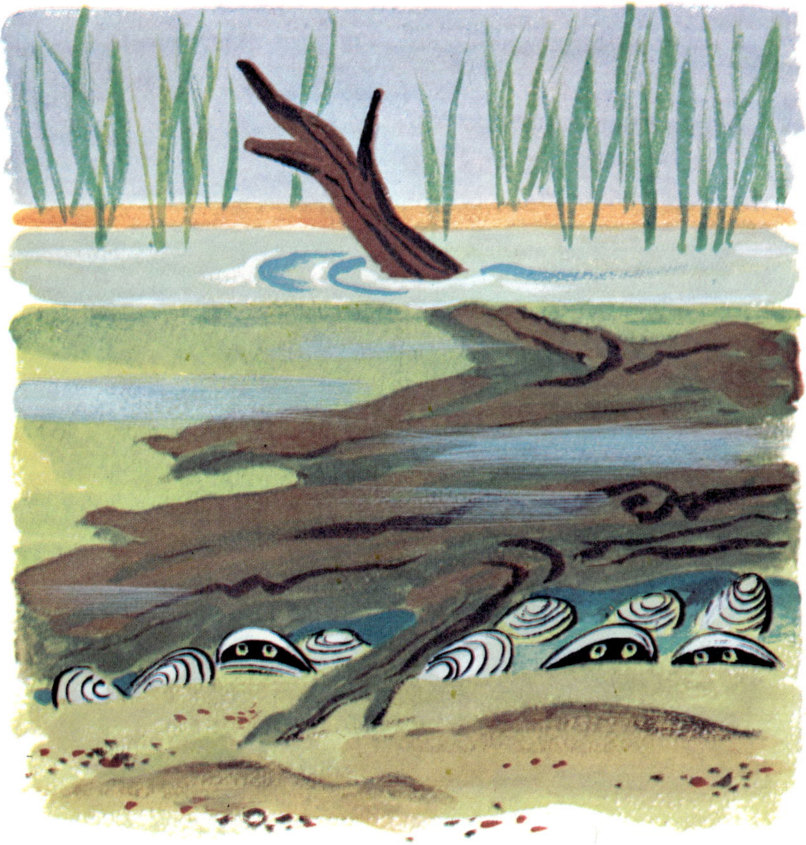

Flat Sam

Ten small clams sat in the sand.
The clams sat under a log.
The water was still and warm.

Clams can dig in the sand.

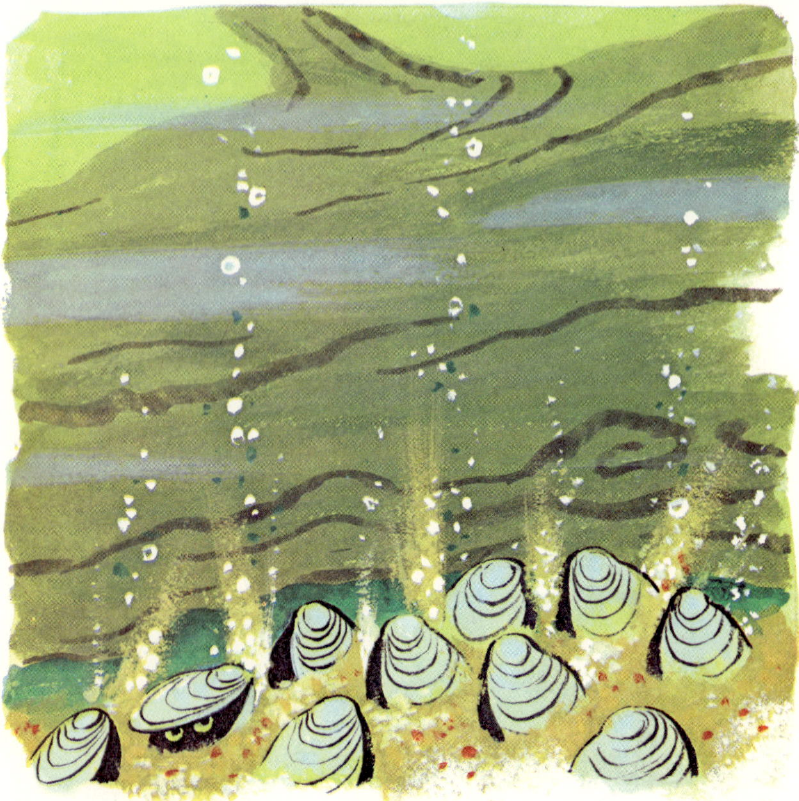

The clams saw Flat Sam.
Flat Sam wanted to get the clams.

A clam called,
"Dig, clams, dig!
Get under the sand!
Dig far into the sand!"

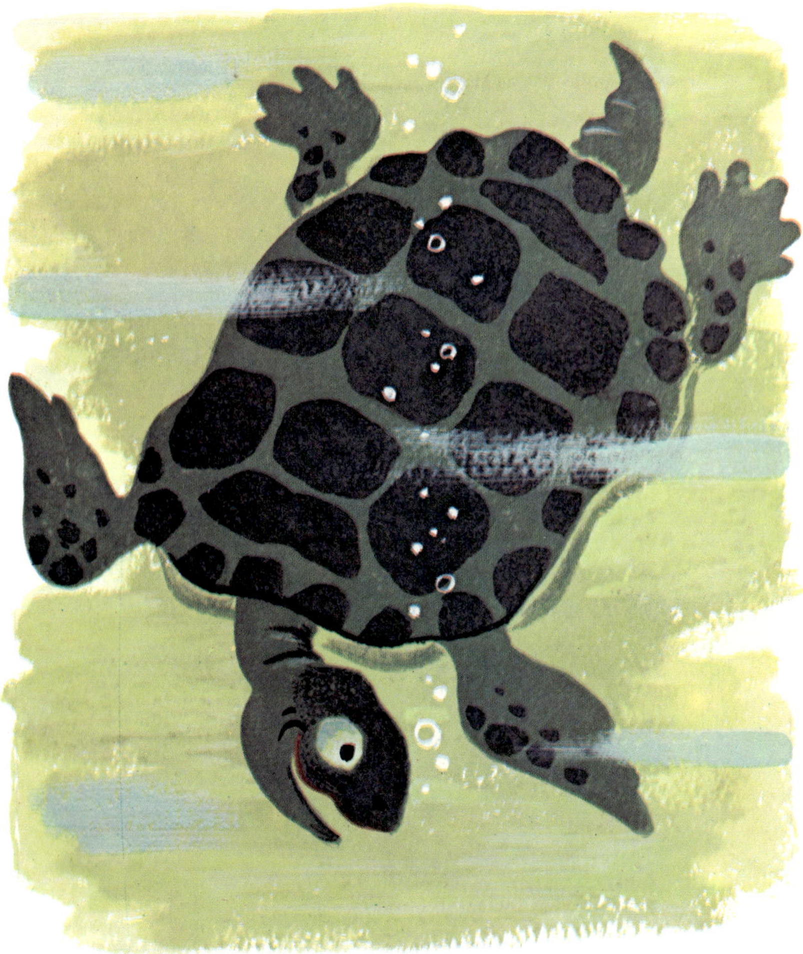

Flat Sam swam after the clams.
The clams dug and dug in the sand.
Will Flat Sam get the clams?

Flat Sam swam fast to the log.

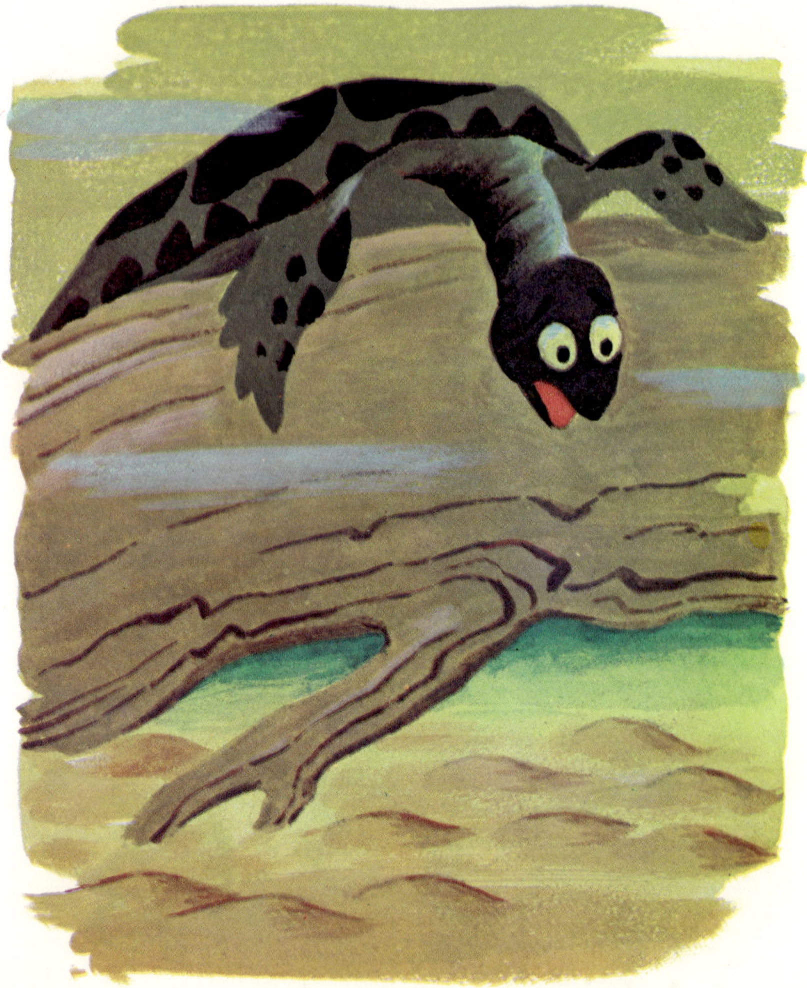

Slap, slap went the water.
Flat Sam did not get the clams.

The small clams were in the sand.
The small clams had dug far down.

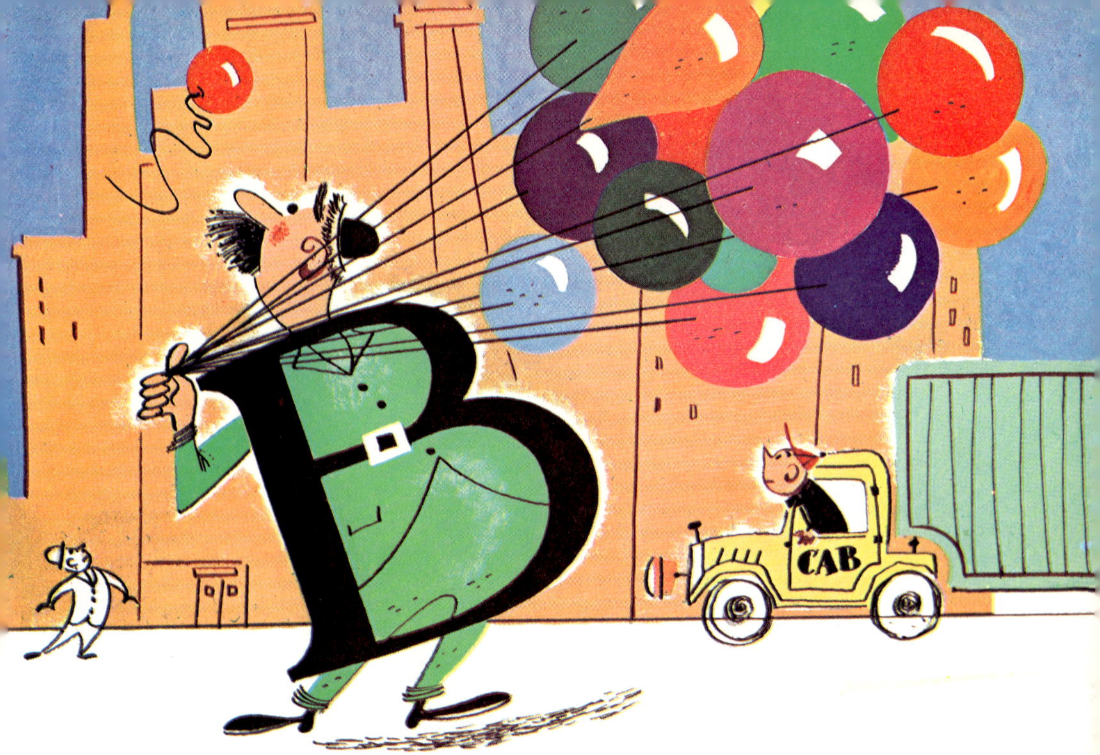

b B

ban bat bar bad Ben best
bed big bin bid beg bond
but bug bog bit barn belt
bass bet bag bald bull bun
ball bend bump bent

rob rub rib tub cob cub
hub slab stub dab cab crab
stab bib bulb Bob Tab

bled blimp blot brim brag number

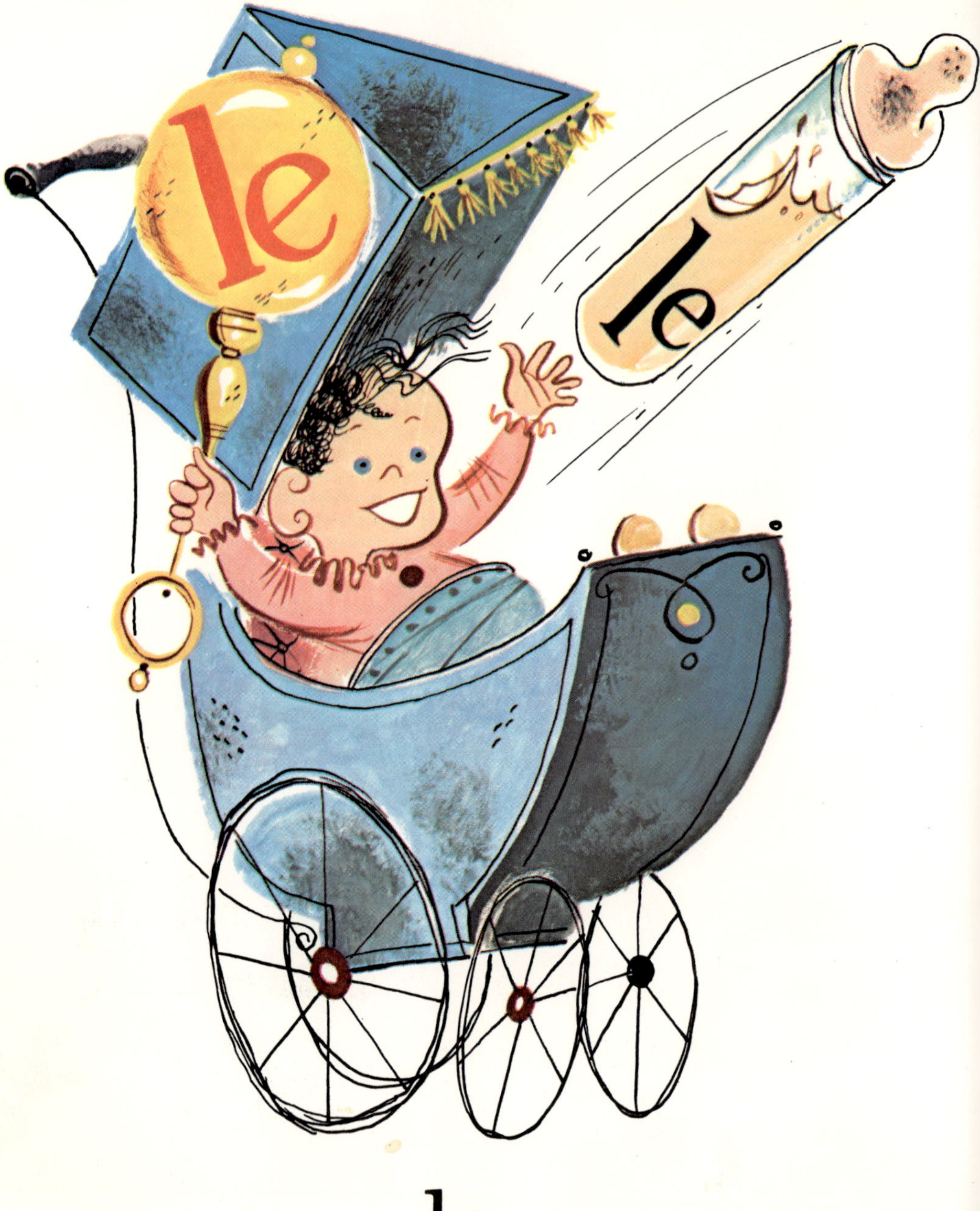

le

bottle little apple rattle
puddle saddle

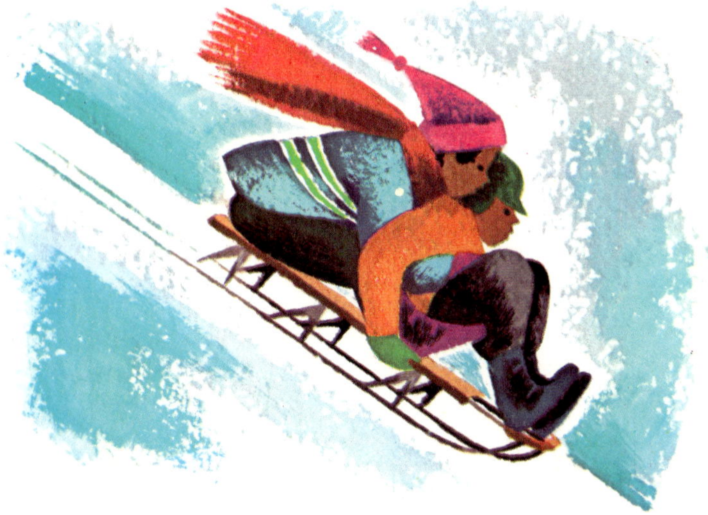

The Little Sled

Bob and Ben sat on a little sled.
The sled started to run fast.
It ran down the big hill.

Faster and faster went the sled.
Bob and Ben held on to it.
"Stop the sled!" said Bob.

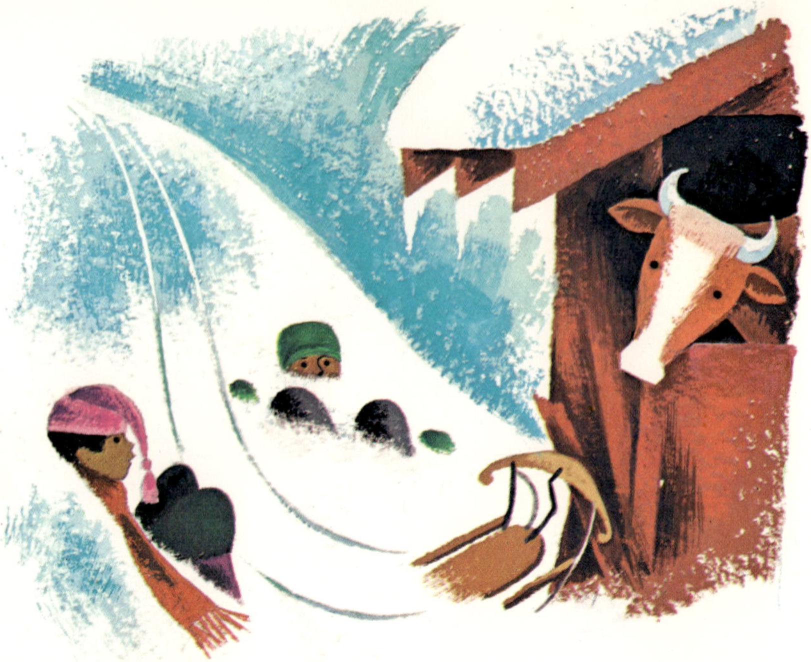

The sled hit a bump.
Bob and Ben fell from the sled.

The little sled did not stop.
It ran on and on.
It ran into a red barn.

The barn bent the little sled.
And the sled dented the barn.

Bob and Ben got wet.

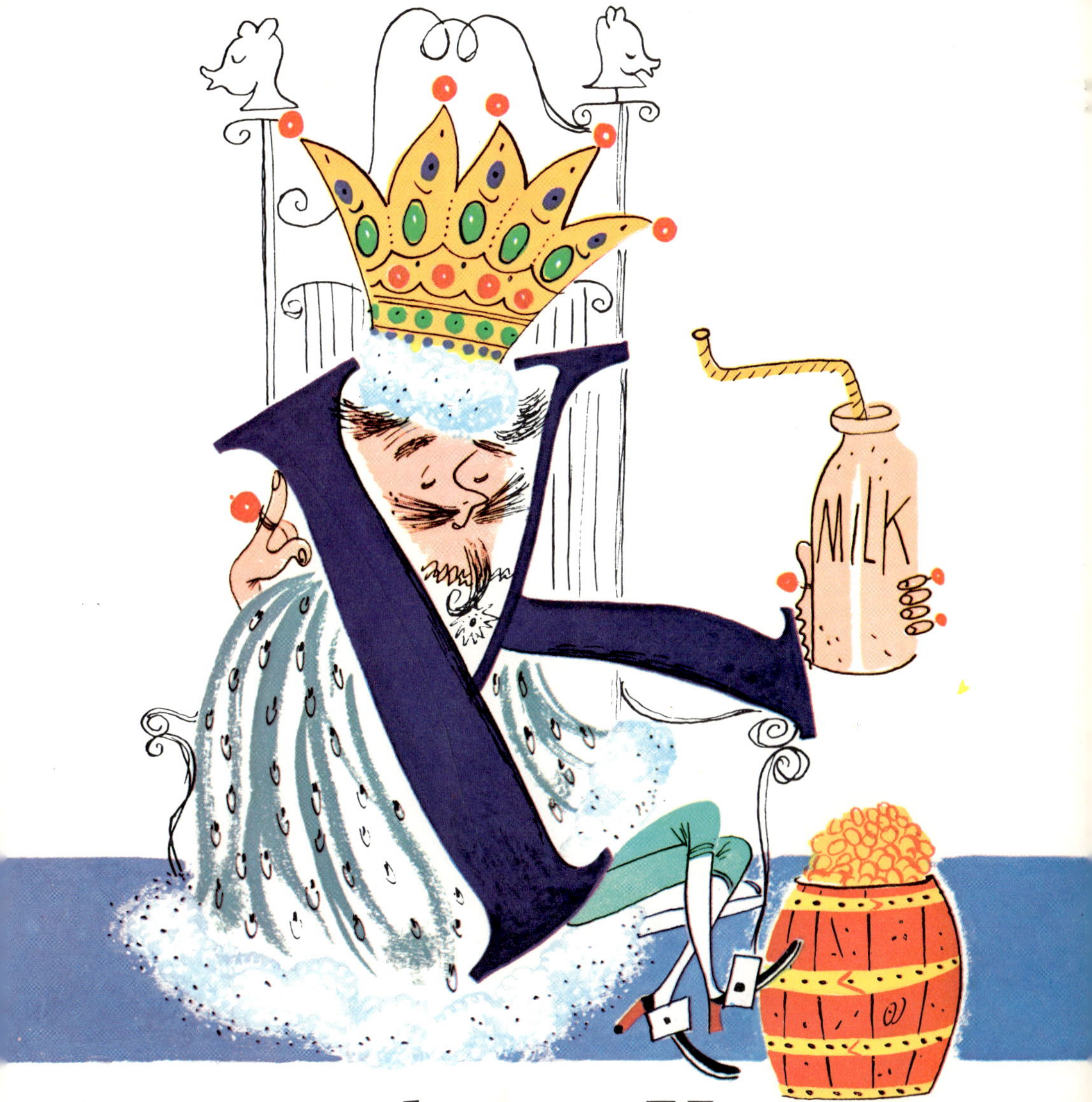

k K

kit kill kept kiss kid keg
milk silk task mask risk brisk
kin dark lark park bark mark
ask kilt kitten

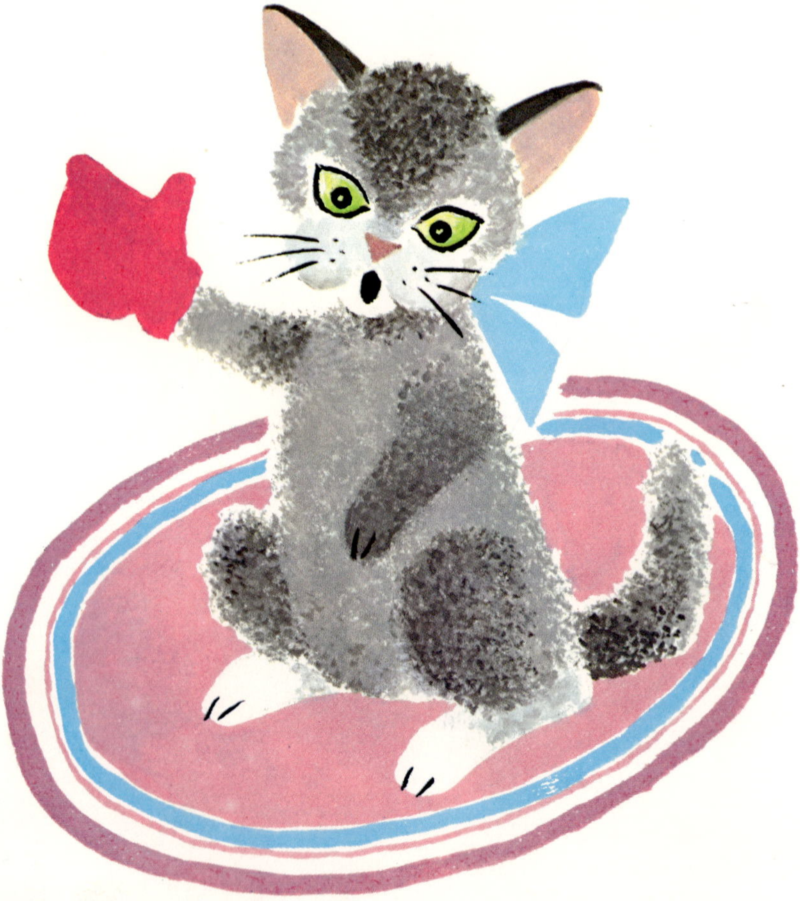

Mitten, mitten
  A mitten on a cat.
Kitten, kitten
  A kitten on a mat.

Adele H. Seronde

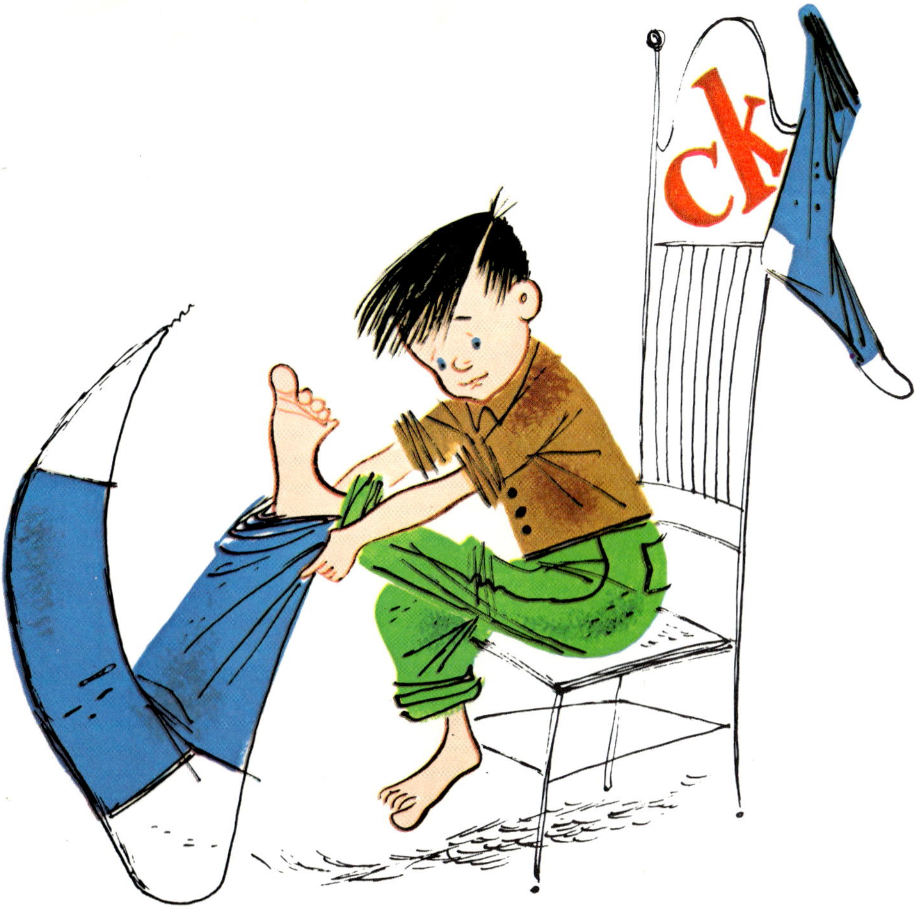

ck

rack sack tack pack lack back
neck deck peck nick sick tick
pick wick lick mock rock sock

dock lock duck luck bucket stack
stick block stuck pluck smack snack
black track truck trick flock kick

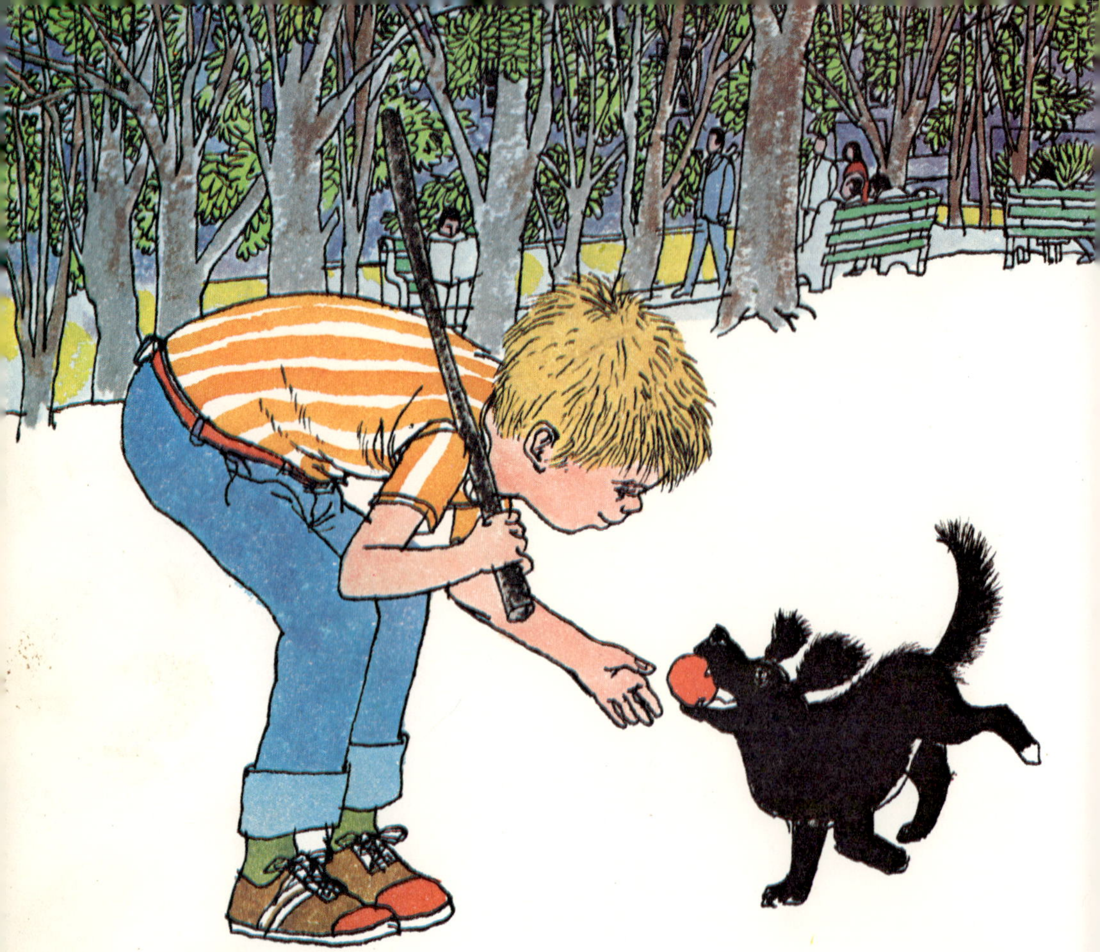

The Little Black Dog

Pick up a stick
And hit the ball—
Hit it across the park.
The little black dog
Will run and run,
And get the ball back and bark!

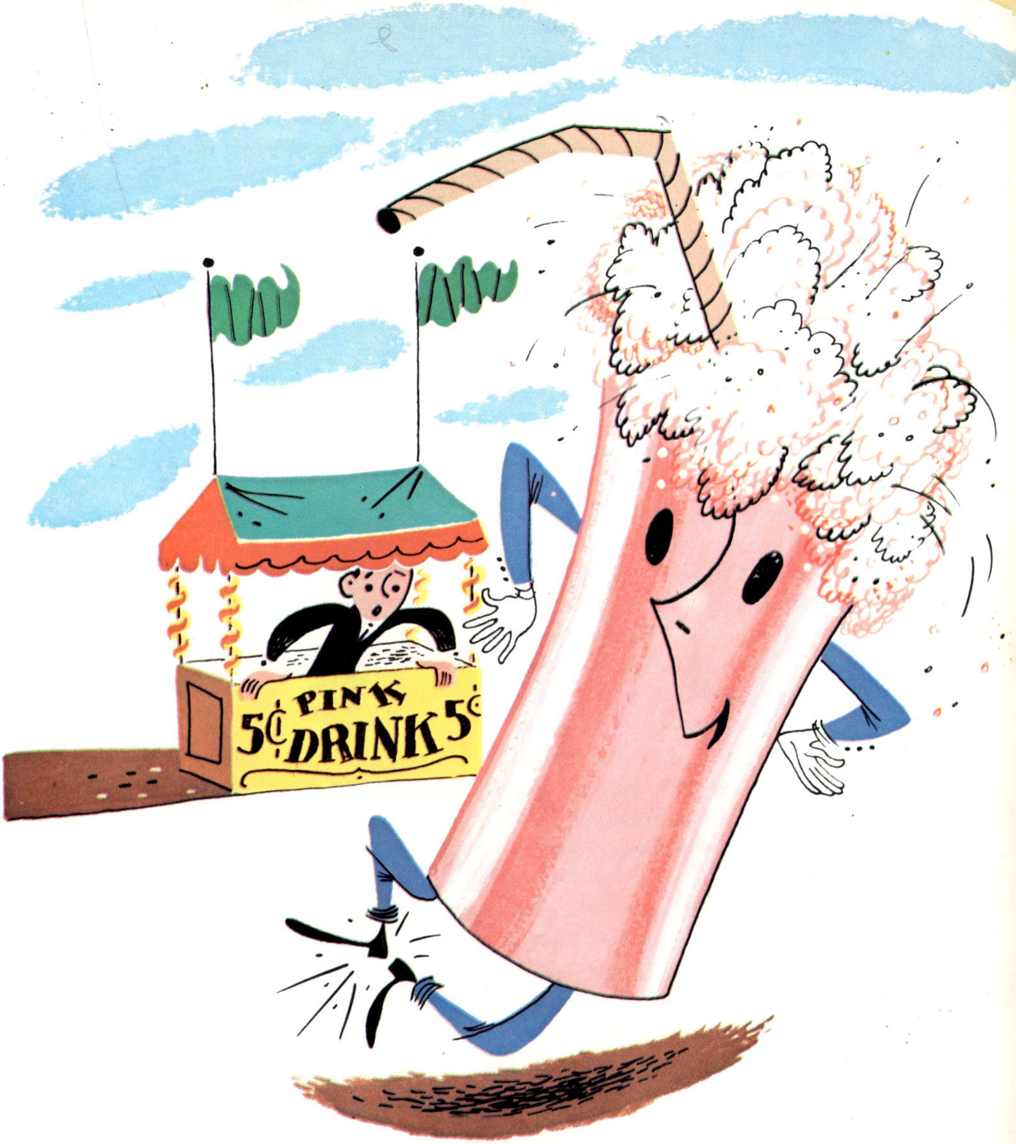

nk

rank	tank	sink	ink	pink
sank	bank	drink	rink	mink
Frank	drank	sunk	link	wink
blanket				

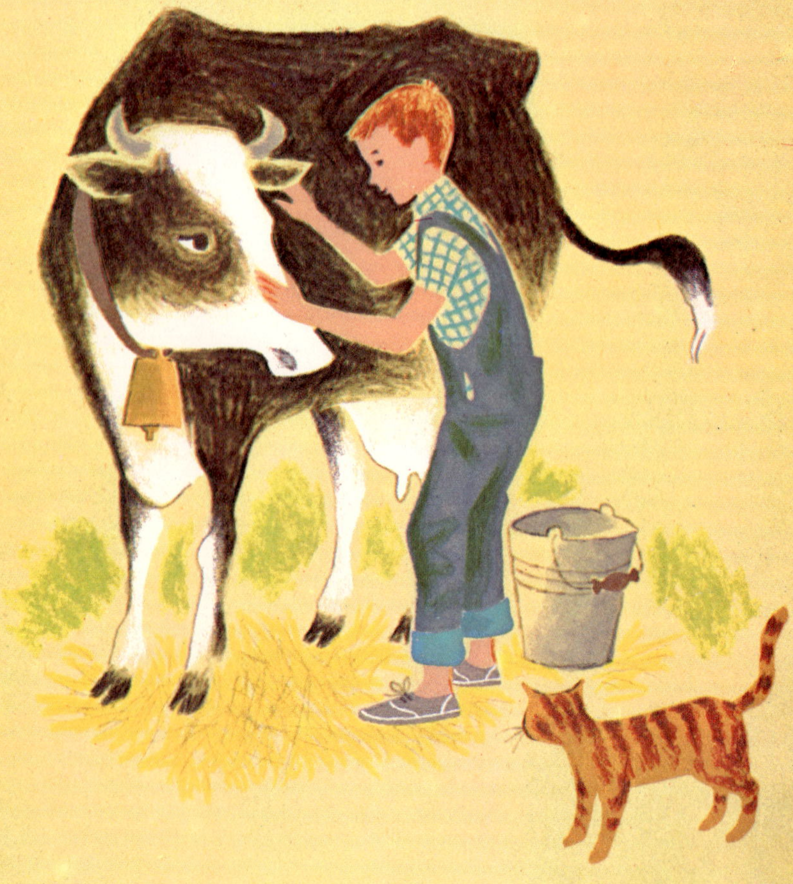

The Black Cow

Bob has a black cow.
The cow is kept in a barn.
Bob rubs her back and neck.
The cow will not harm Bob.

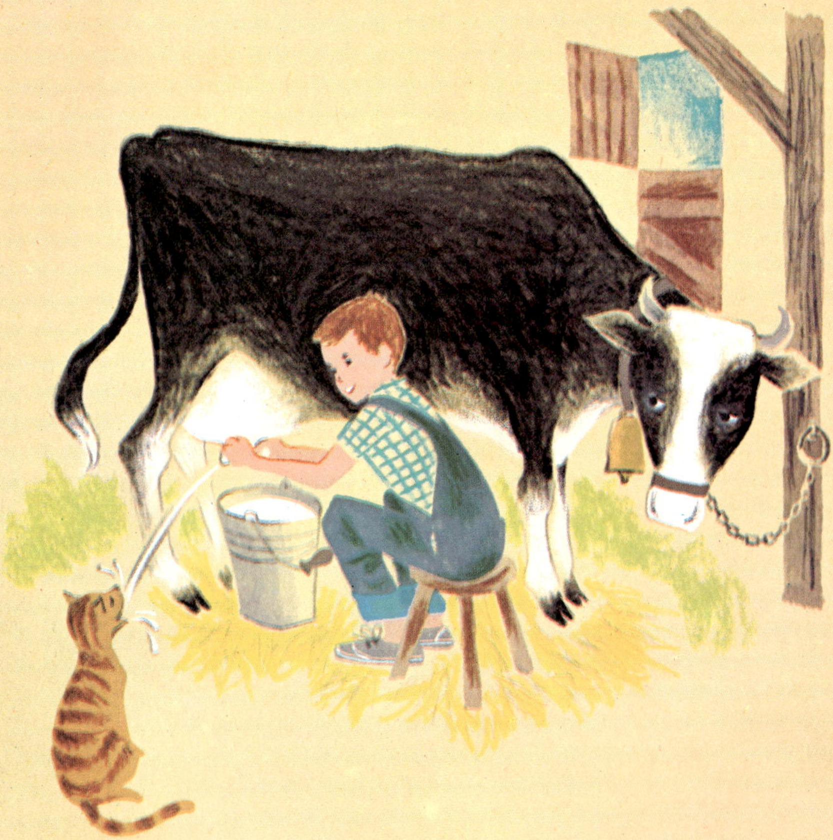

Bob wants to get milk.
Bob can milk his black cow.

Tab is a tan cat.
The cat begs for a drink of milk.
Bob milks the cow for Tab.

of

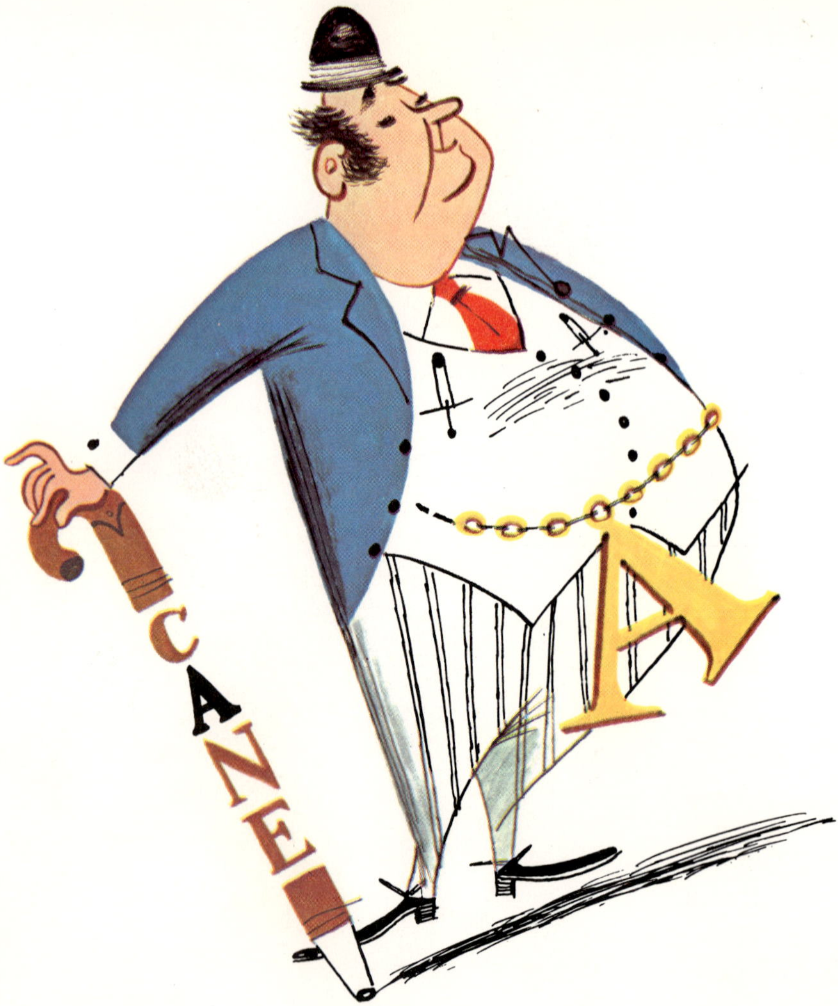

a-e

can	cane	mat	mate
at	ate	fat	fate
rat	rate	man	mane
cap	cape	pan	pane

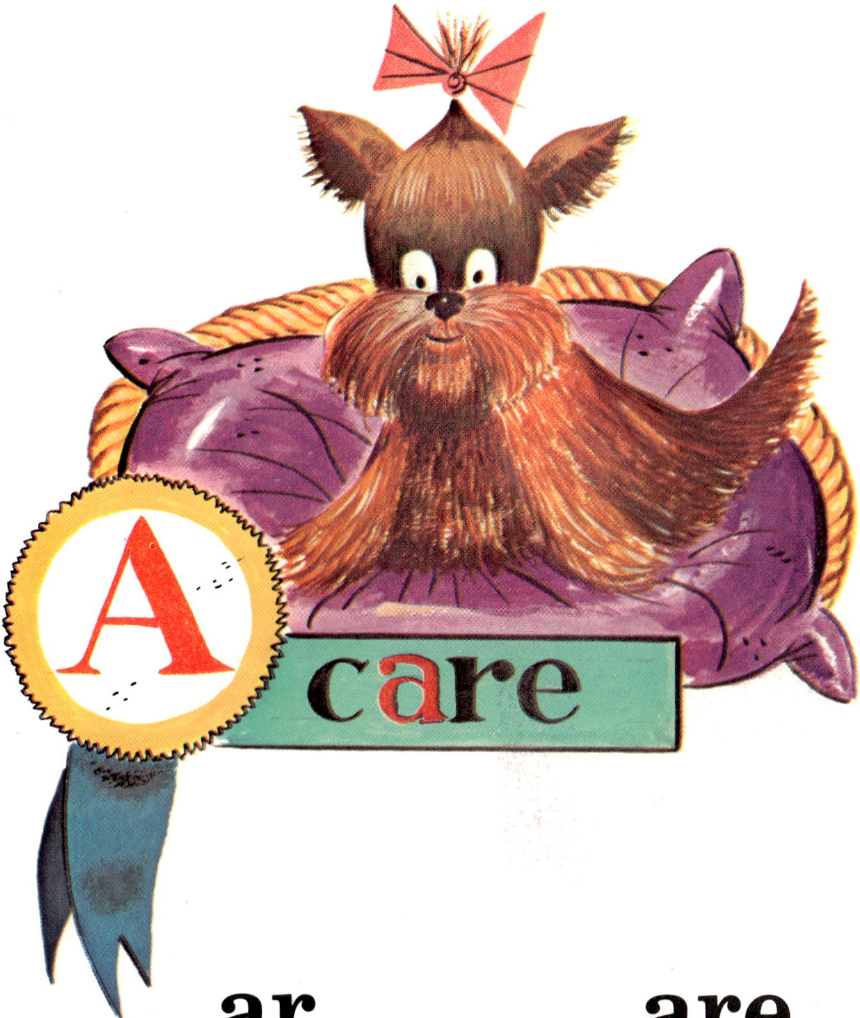

ar **are**

car	care	bar	bare
mar	mare	star	stare
far	fare	scar	scare

dare hare ware flare

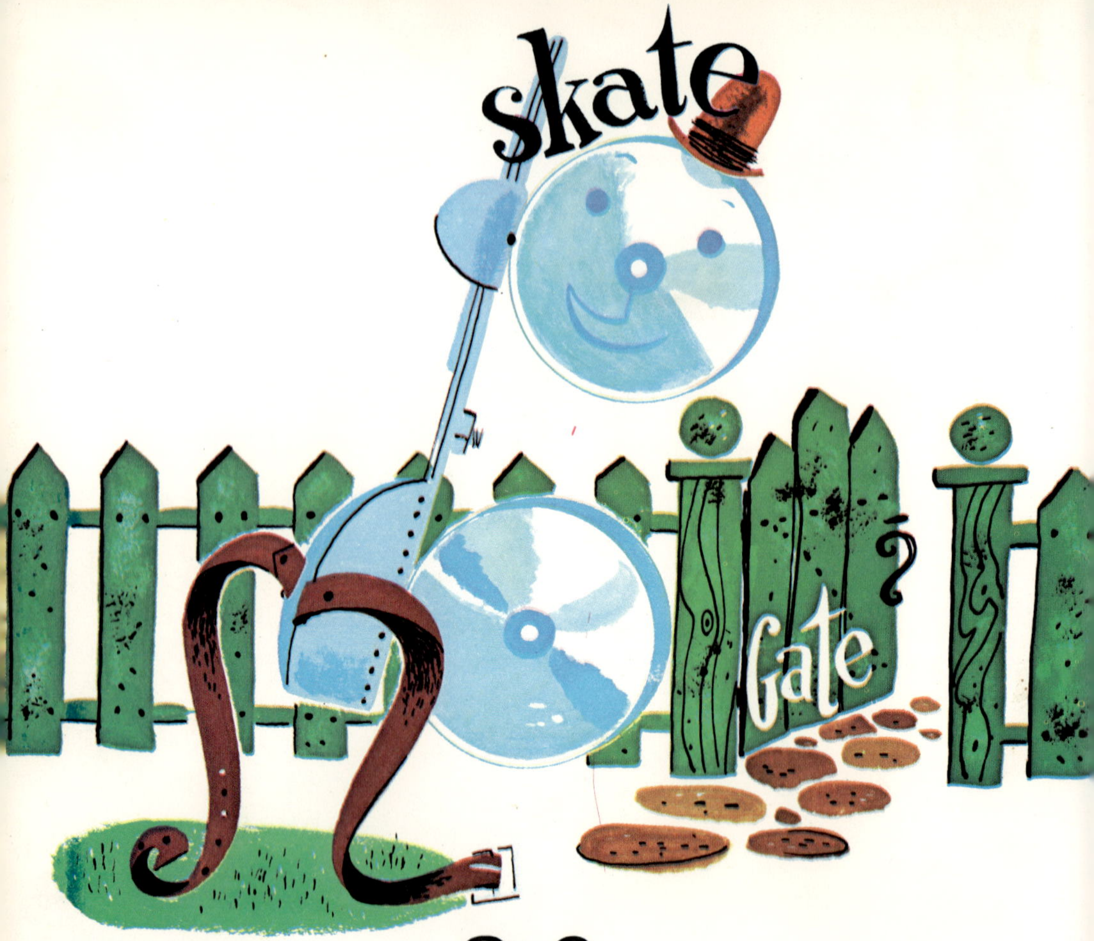

a-e

name late Kate safe base bake
tale date blame make sake lake
taste same came wake made spade

gale bale stale take sale hate
gate state grate game pale cake
plane tame skate rake snake

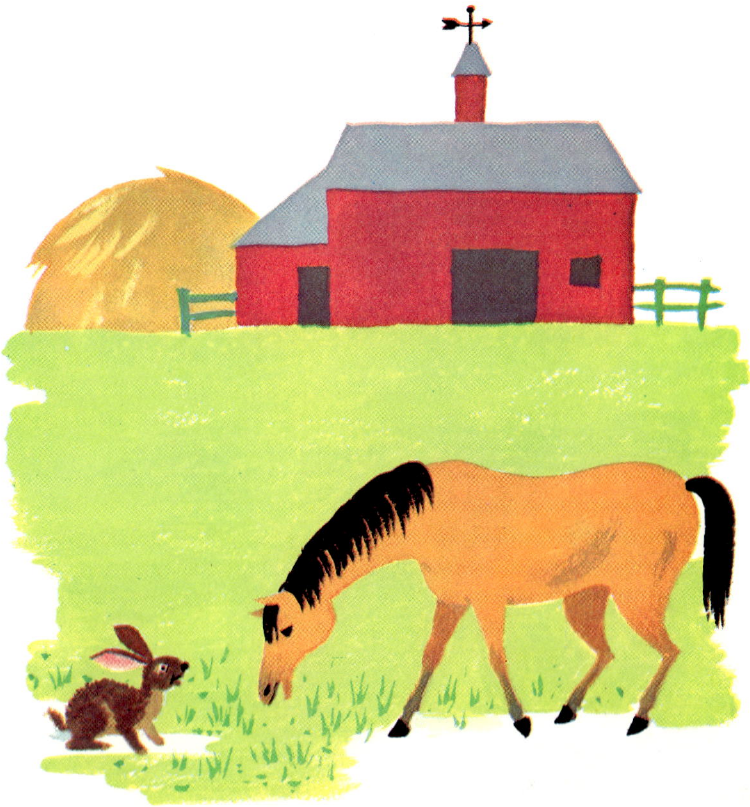

Black Mane and Tim

Black Mane was a pet mare.
Her mane was black as slate.

Tim was a small, brown hare.

Black Mane and Tim ate grass.

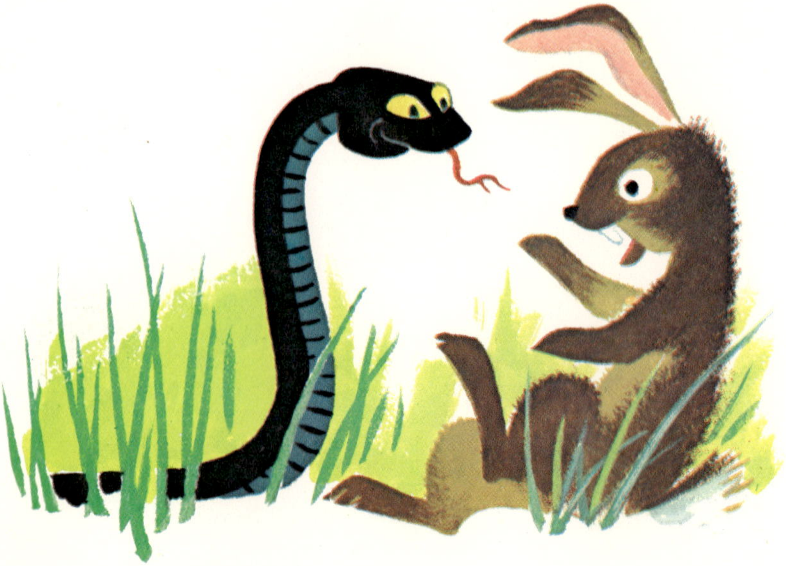

Tim saw a snake in the grass.
The snake came up to Tim.
Tim saw the snake stare at him.
It was a big, black snake.

Black Mane ran to the gate.
Tim was on her back.
Tim made Black Mane run fast.
"Run, Black Mane, run!" said Tim.

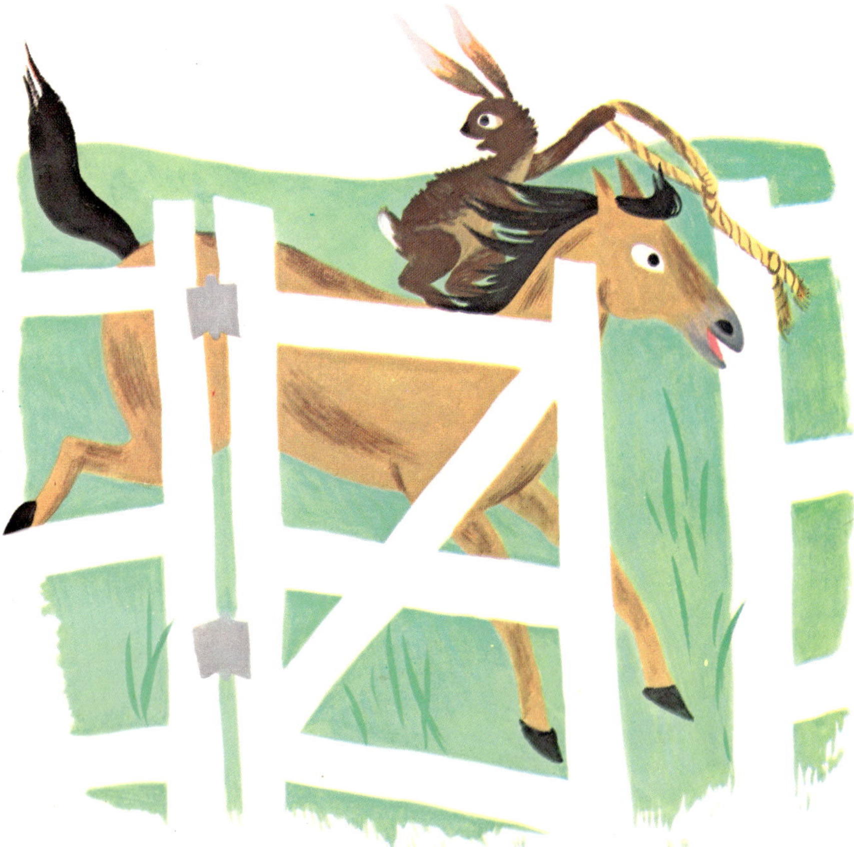

Black Mane came to the gate.
It was as tall as the mare.
"Help, Tim!" said Black Mane.

Tim helped Black Mane.
Black Mane helped Tim.
The snake did not get the hare.

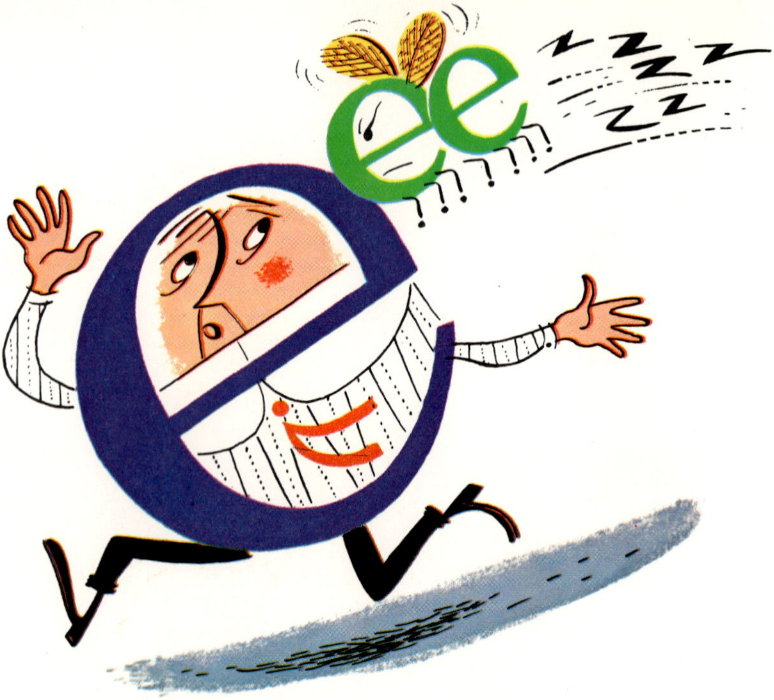

e E ee

he be me we Pete here

bee see seem seed seek steel
flee beet beef meet deer reel
deep keep peek peel feel tree

feed feet need sleep week street
deeper feeler keeper fifteen green

been

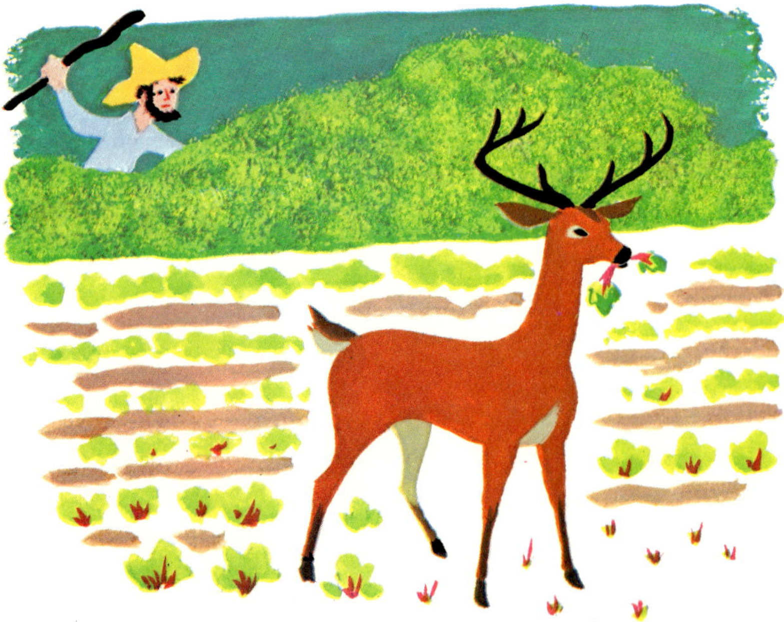

Red Deer

Red Deer went to a beet farm.
He wanted to feed on the beets.
The deer did not see the farmer.
The farmer did not want Red Deer to nip the tops off his beets.
The beet farmer hid under a tree.
He had a stick.

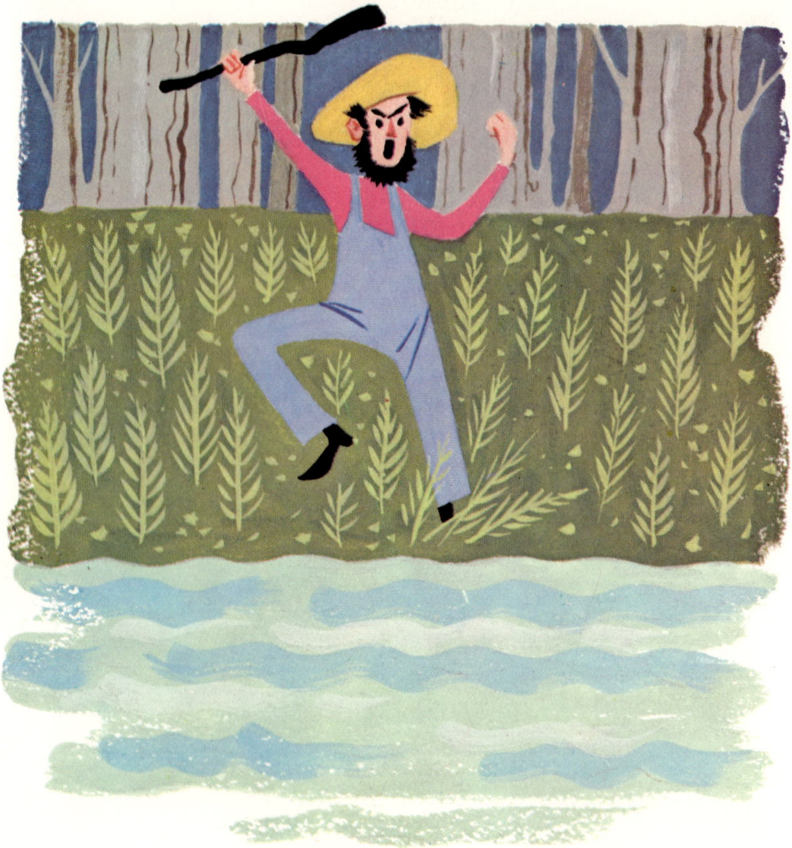

The farmer picked up the stick and started after Red Deer.

Red Deer ran down a steep hill. He hid in the deep grass. But the farmer saw his antlers.

Red Deer swam across the deep water.

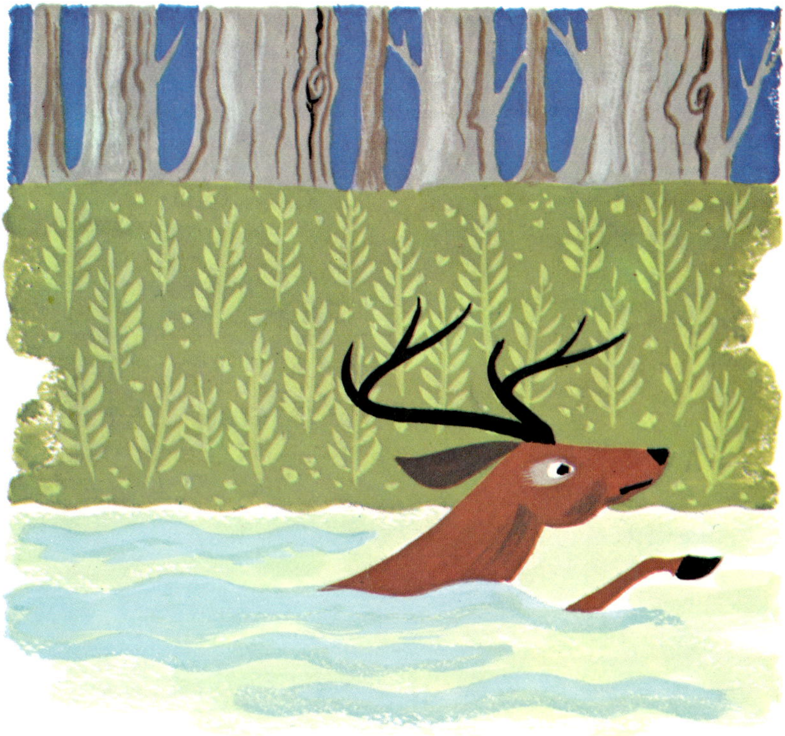

He ran into the tall trees.

The farmer did not hit him.

Red Deer will not be back to the beet farm.

He will not nip the tops off the beets.

He will feed in the forest and be safe from the farmer.

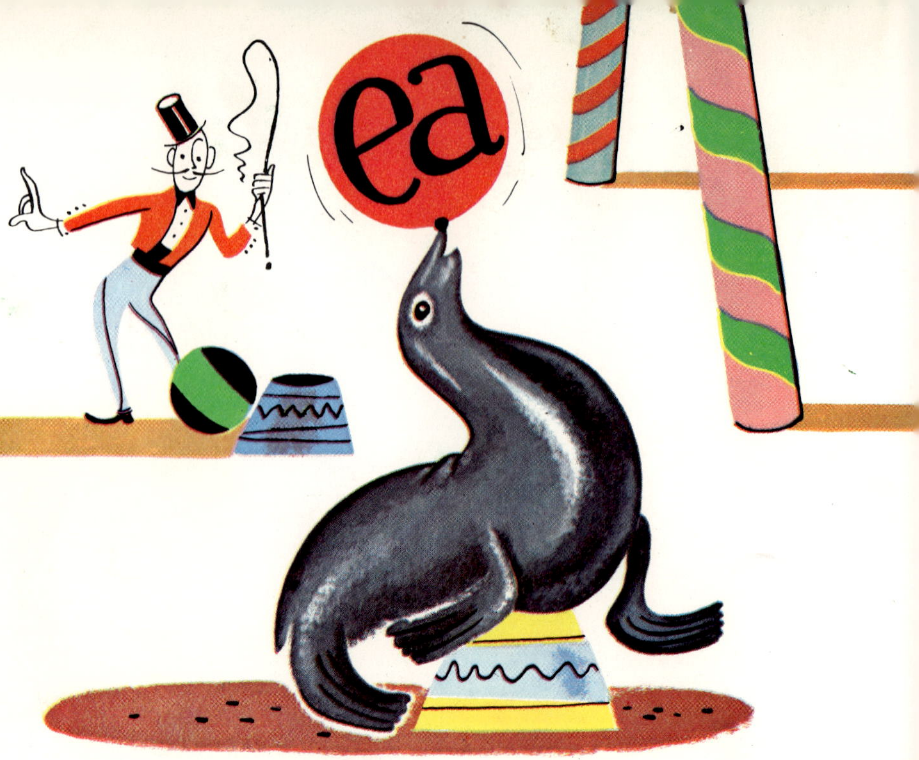

ea

ear bean leak meat reap neat
eat fear lean pea seam read

east feast leap peak seat near
ease heat lease tea bead beak
beat heal least seal team please

beam leaf meal rear tease beard
beast lead mean sea dear pleat
repeat retreat steam defeat

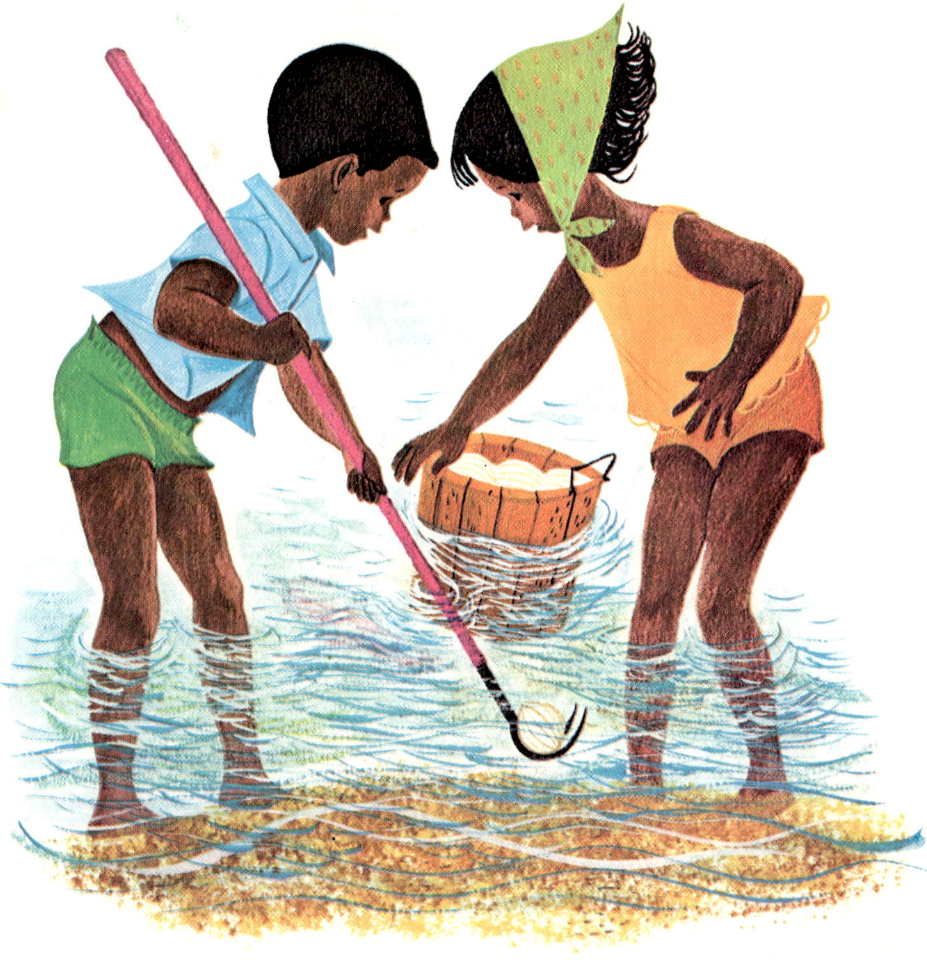

Don and Nell Dig Clams

Don and Nell went to the sea to dig clams.

Nell wanted clams to eat.

Don had a bucket and a rake on the end of a stick.

He and Nell dug for clams.

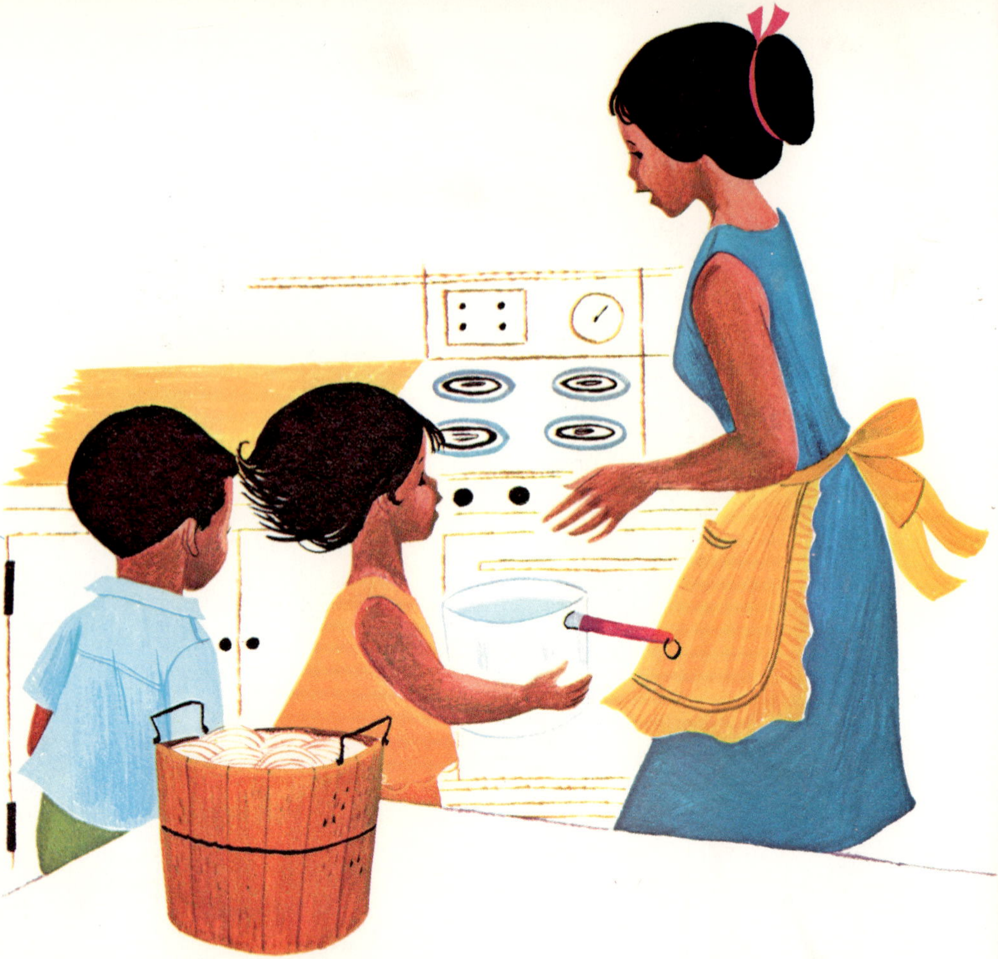

"We will steam the clams," said Don.

"I will heat the water," said Nell.

Don and Nell steamed the bucket of clams.

I

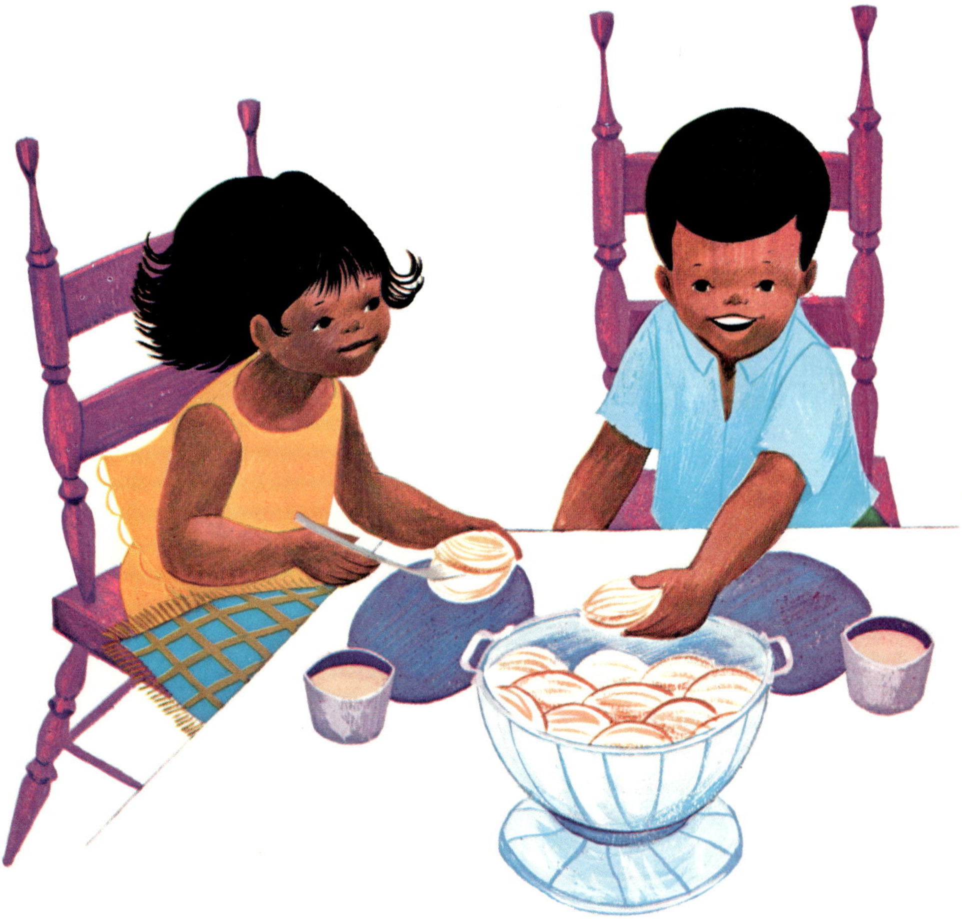

“Please pass me a clam,” said Nell.

Nell ate ten clams for her meal. Don ate fifteen clams.

After the big meal, Don and Nell were full of clams.

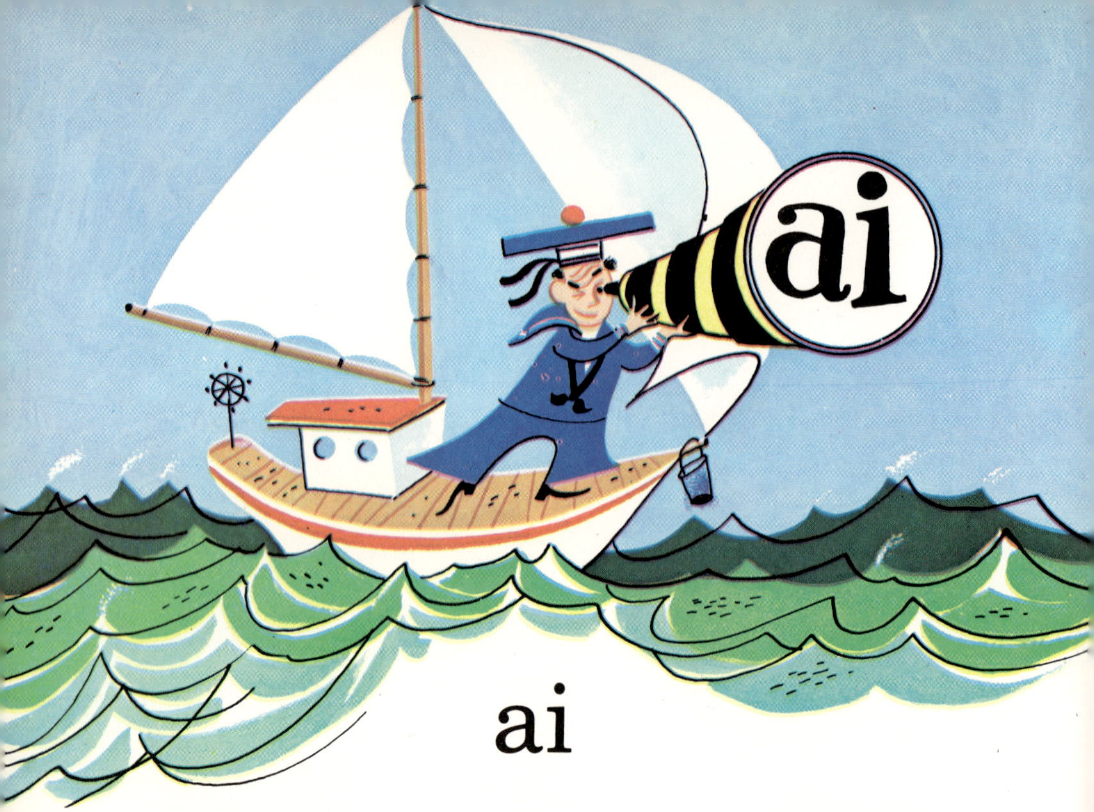

ai

aim claim rain gain main grain
drain brain train faint maid paid
braid fail rail hail mail tail
Gail raise waist

air hair pair

sail pain Spain gait slain stain
plain pail nail bait wait trailer
afraid sprain praise strain paint

again

An ant
Will pass
In a forest
Of grass
On a twig
Near a rain-
Puddle
Sea.
And a rock
Will be
A hill
Tip-top
And a fern
A monster
Tree.

Adele H. Seronde

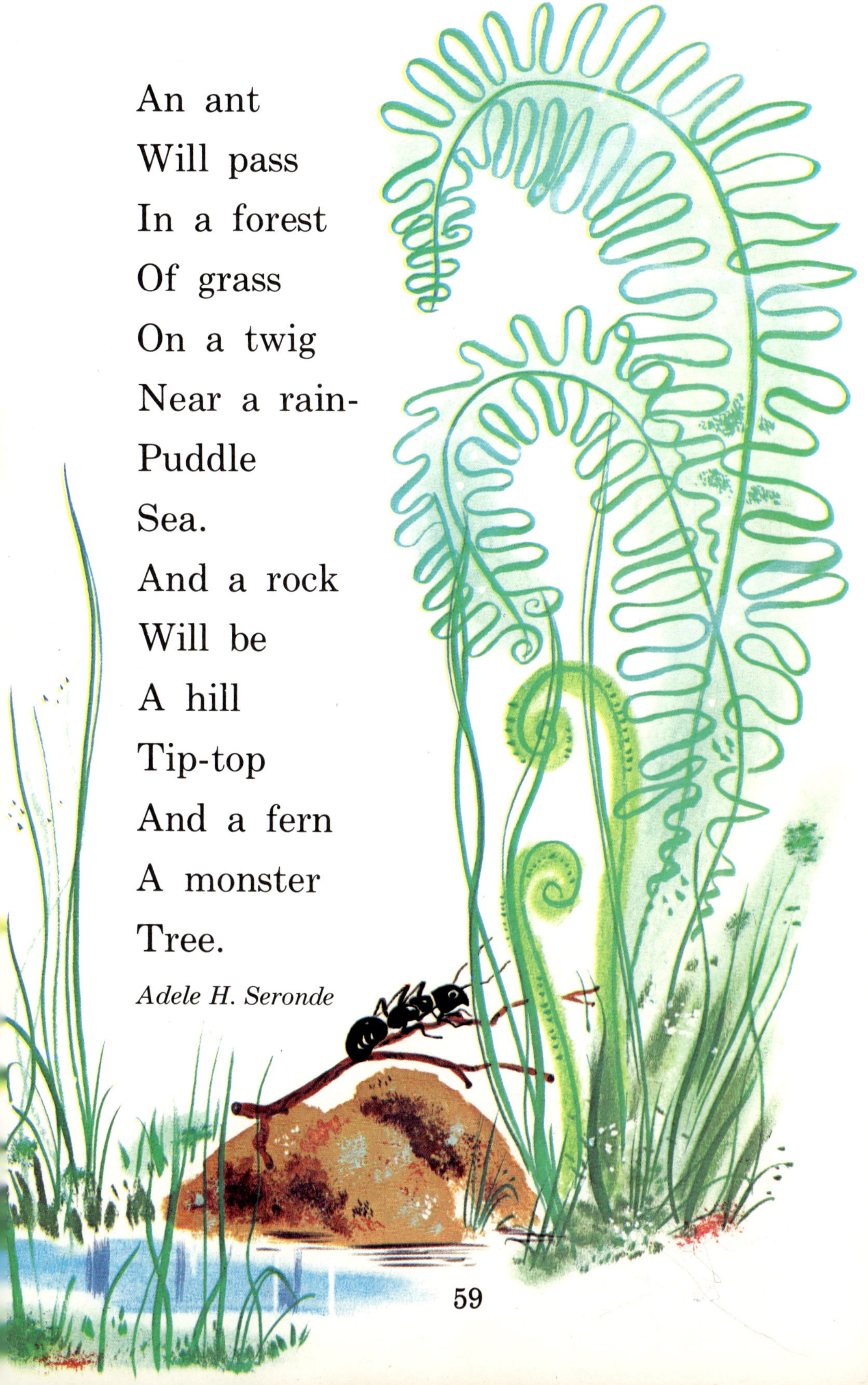

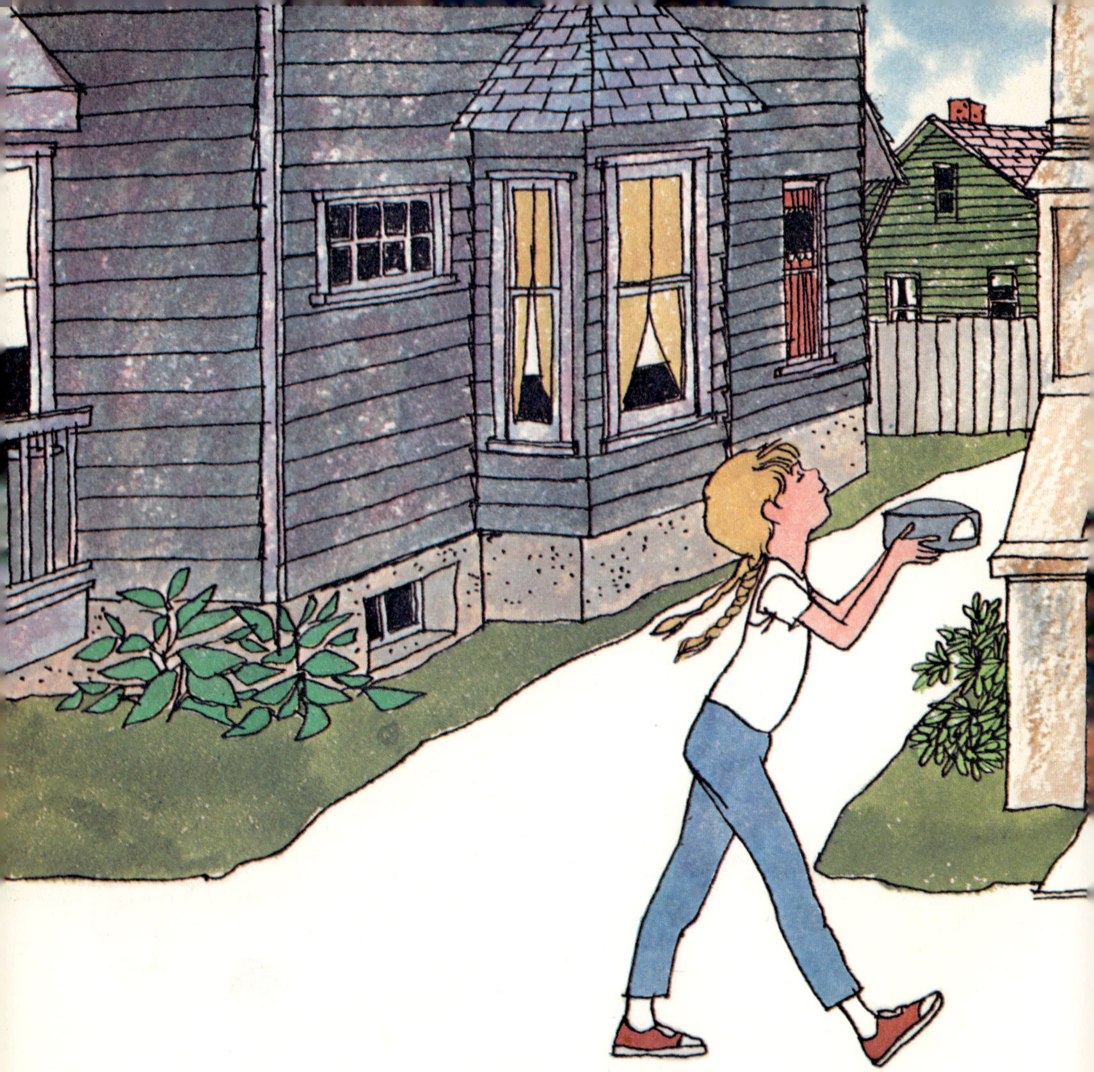

The Mail Carrier

The town mail carrier said, "I need help to deliver the mail."

"I can help," said Gail.

"Please, can I help?" asked Kate.

carrier deliver

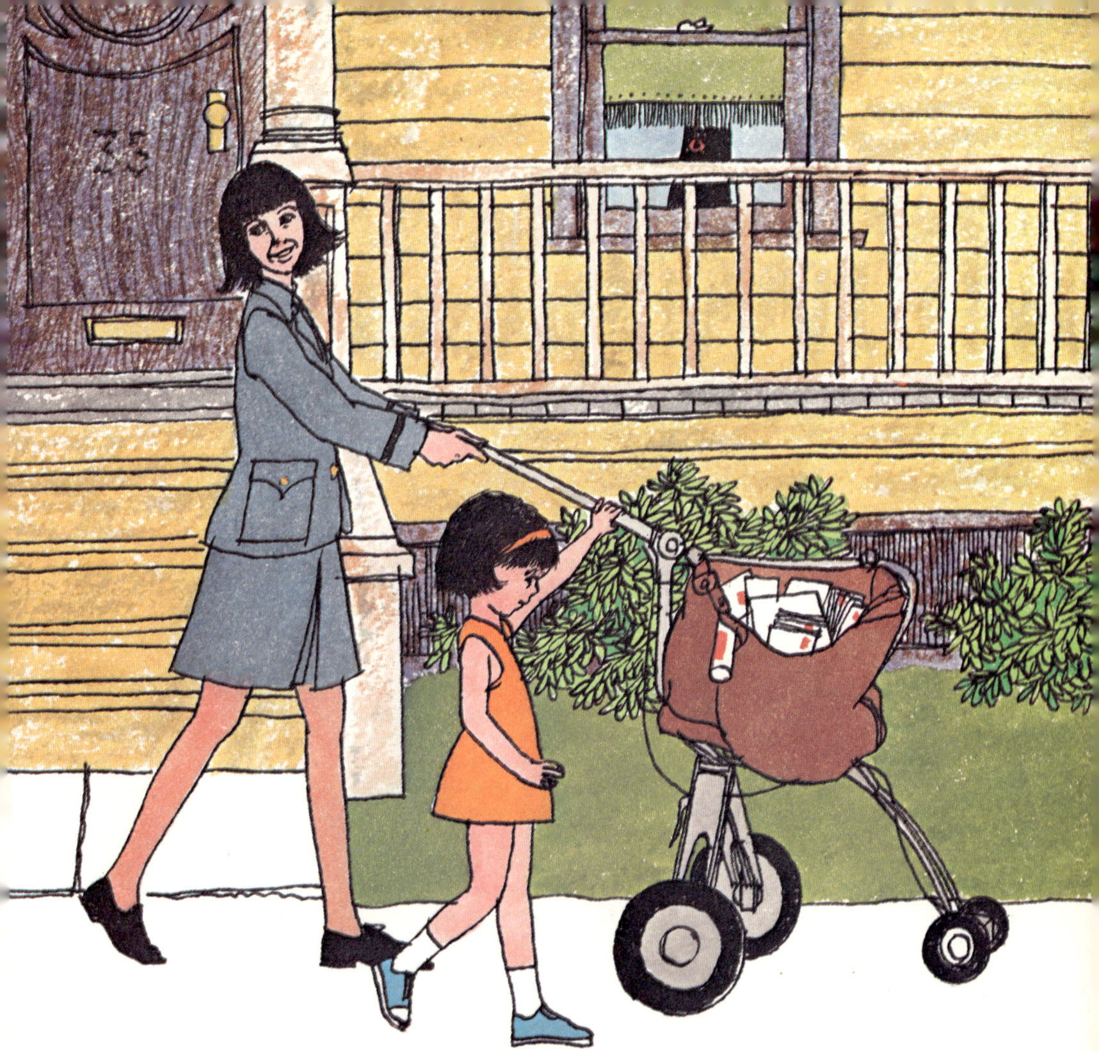

Gail held her cap. Kate put her hand on the mail cart.

The mail carrier said, "It's hard to deliver the mail fast. Lots of numbers are hard to see. The numbers need to be painted again."

"Here is a letter from Spain," said the mail carrier.

"It is for Frank Green. The address is 15 Main Street. But I did not see a number fifteen on Main Street."

"I can help," said Kate.

"Let me help, too," said Gail.

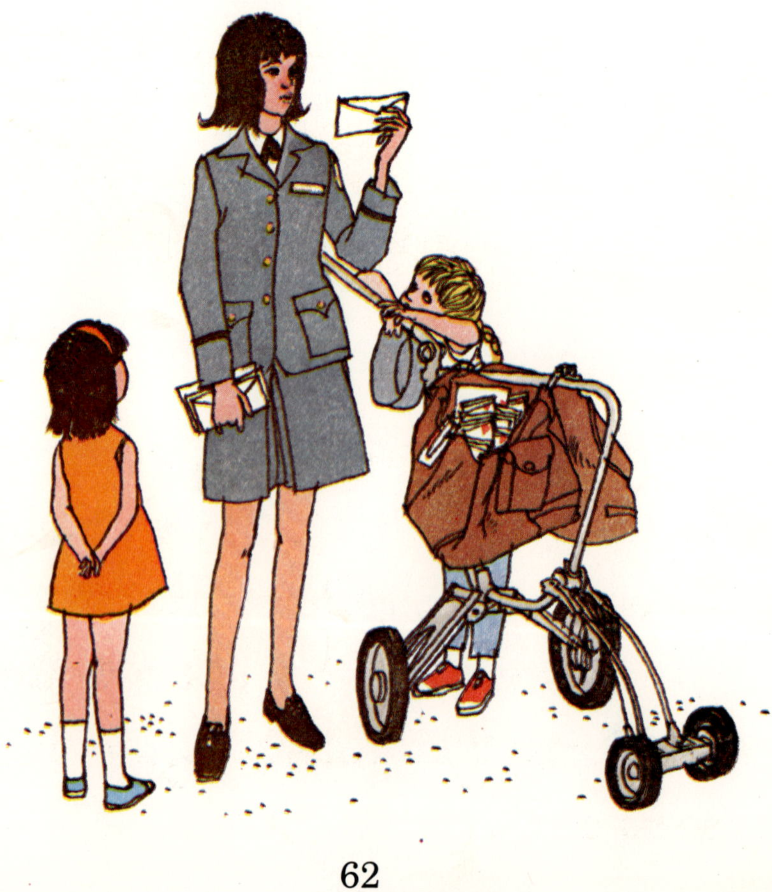

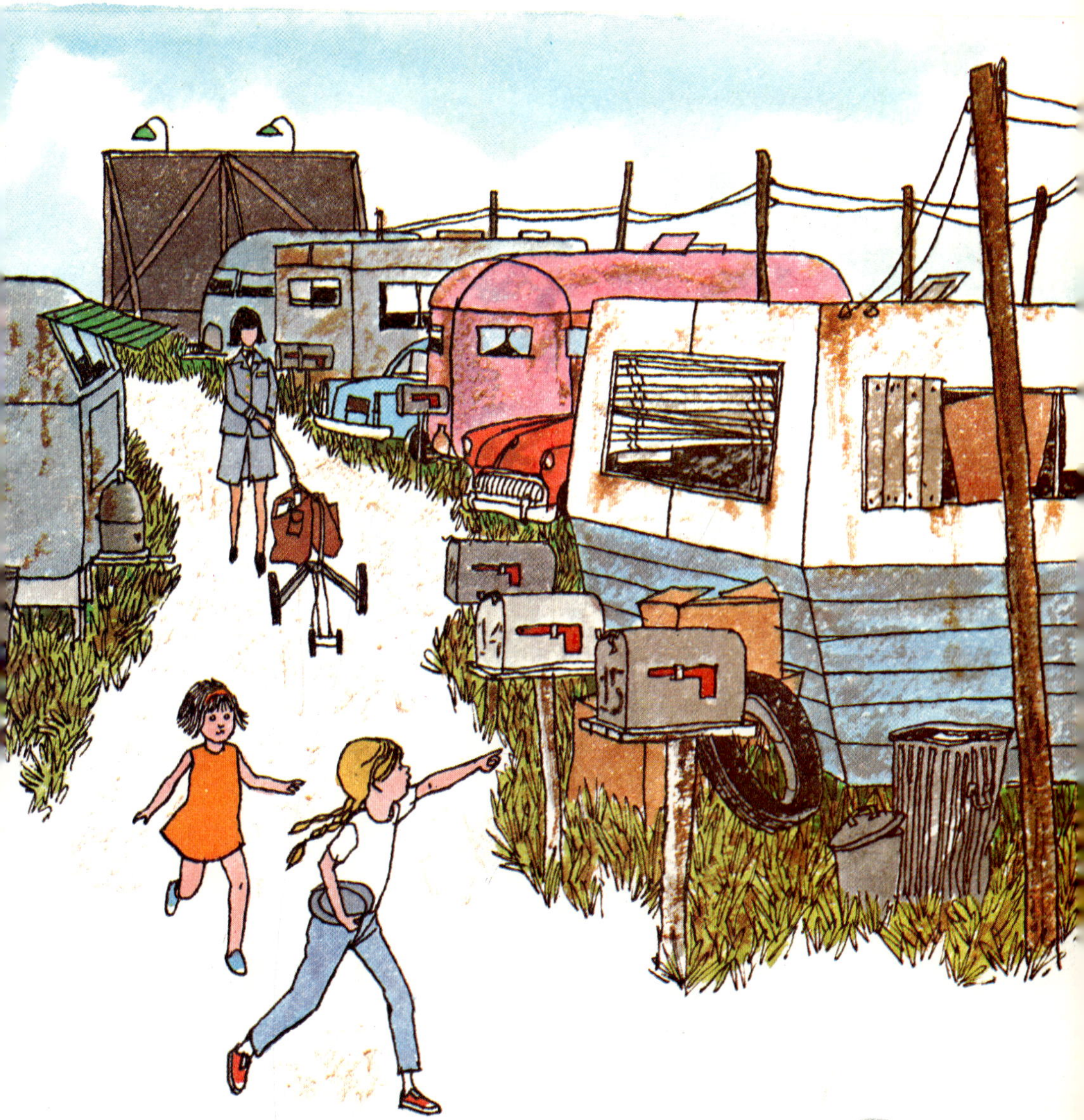

"Frank Green is in a trailer on Main Street. His trailer is number fifteen in the trailer park."

The mail carrier praised Gail and Kate and said, "Please help me again."

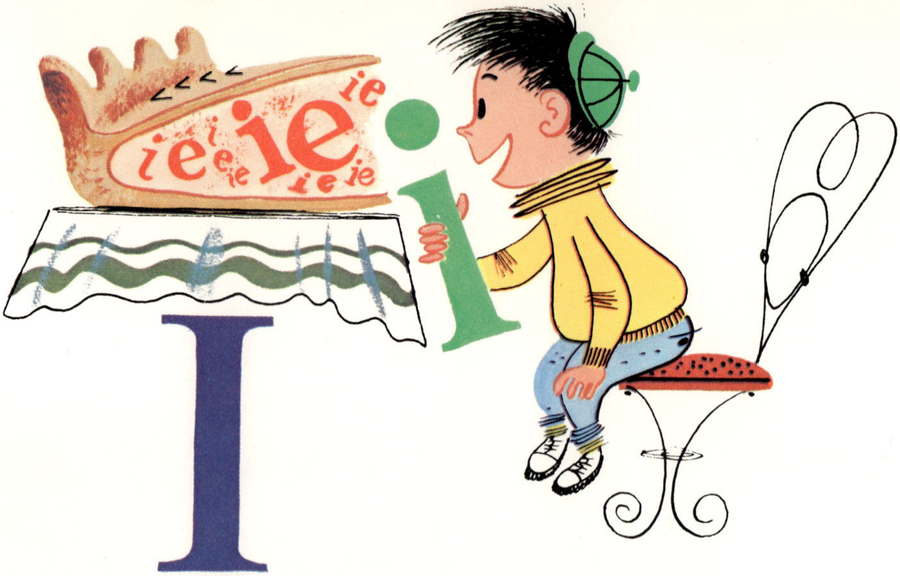

i I ie

mine ride pile Mike bite spike
pine side bike tile dime strike
nine hide time like pipe spite

fine wide life stile smile bride
line ripe mile lime stride diner
kite wife spine dike crime finer

find kind mind bind behind pilot

tie lie die pie cried dried tried

ir

sir fir first bird girl dirt

sire fire spire hire tire

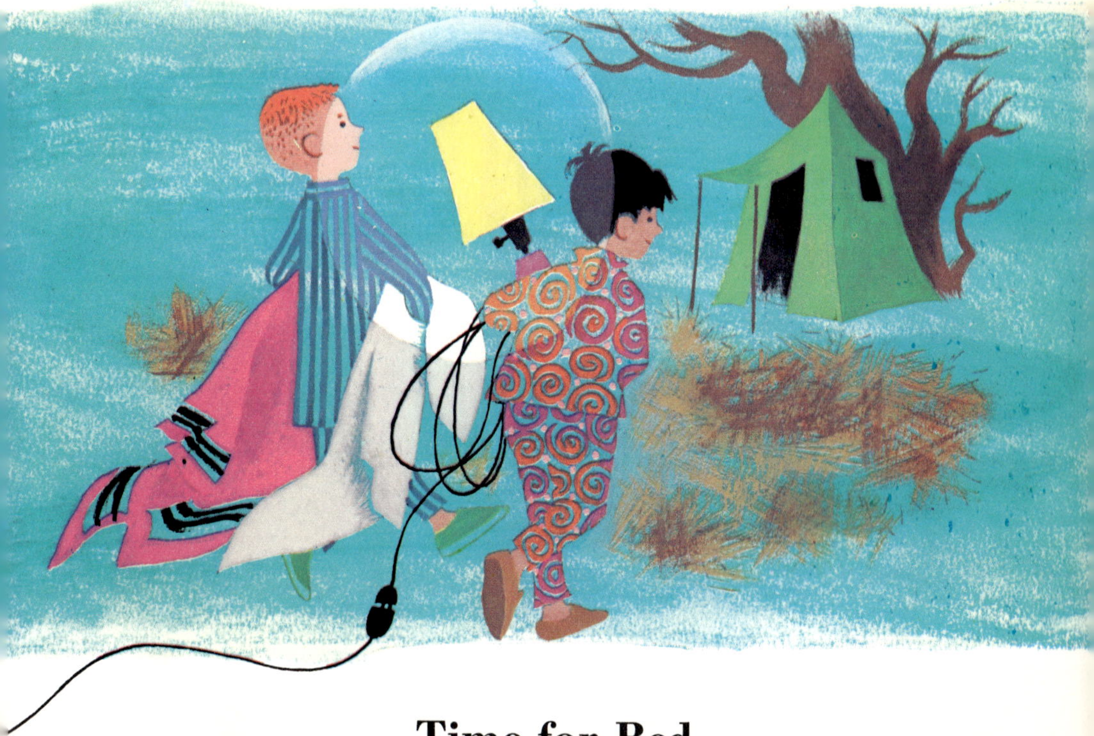

Time for Bed

It is time for Bill and Mike to be in bed.

"I like to be in bed at nine," said Bill.

"I will be in bed first."

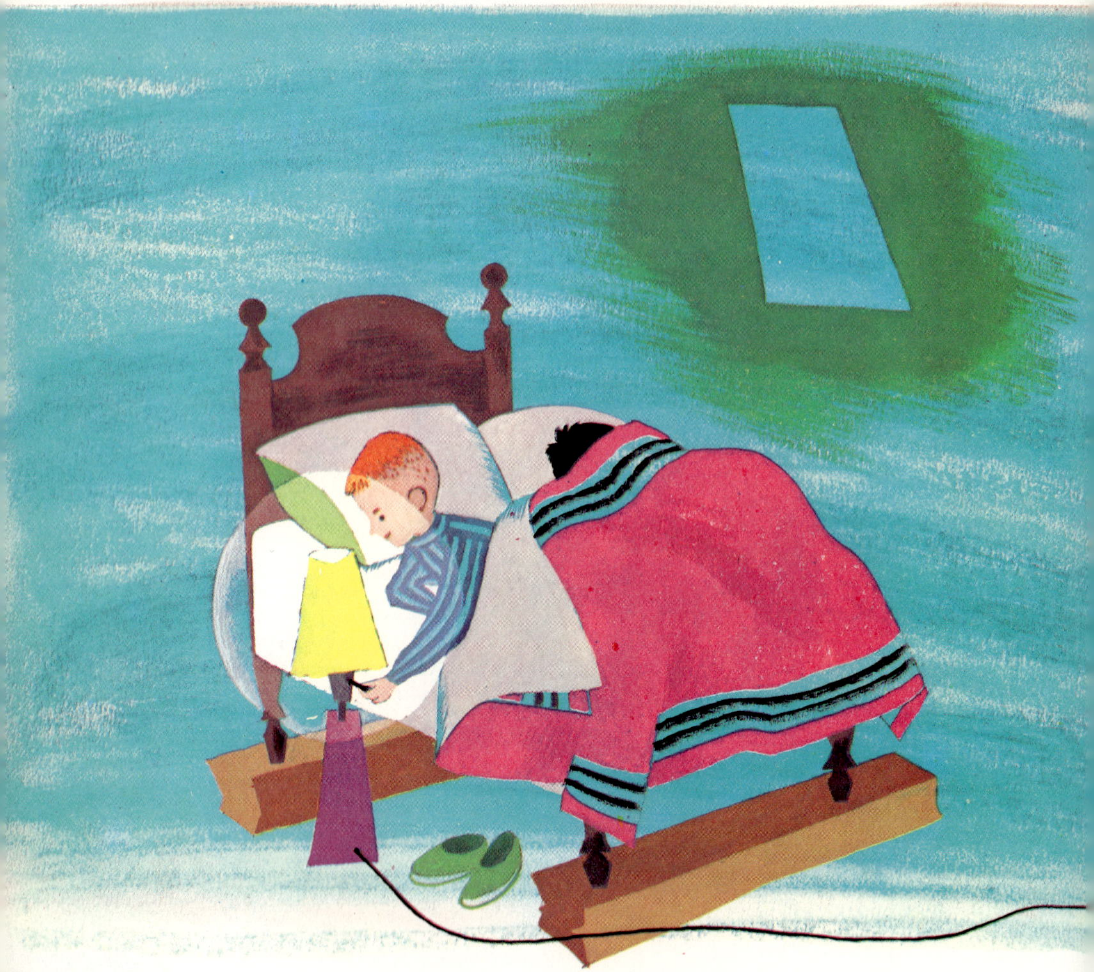

Mike snapped off the lamp.

Mike and Bill had a fine bed in a tent.

It was a big, wide bed.

It was raised on a pair of blocks.

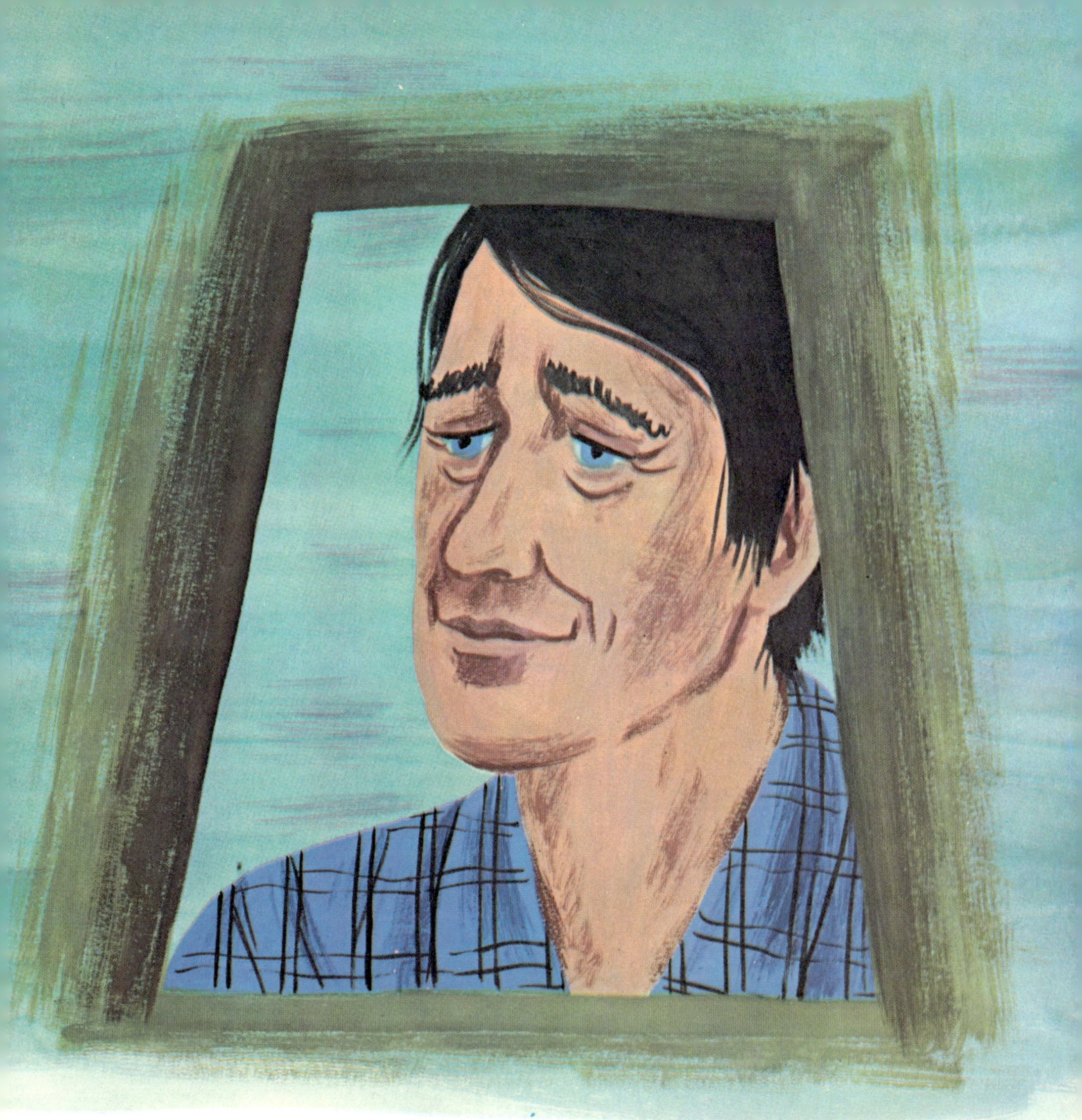

"I see a man," cried Bill.

"Hide under the blanket.
I am afraid."

Mike and Bill hid under the red and black blanket.

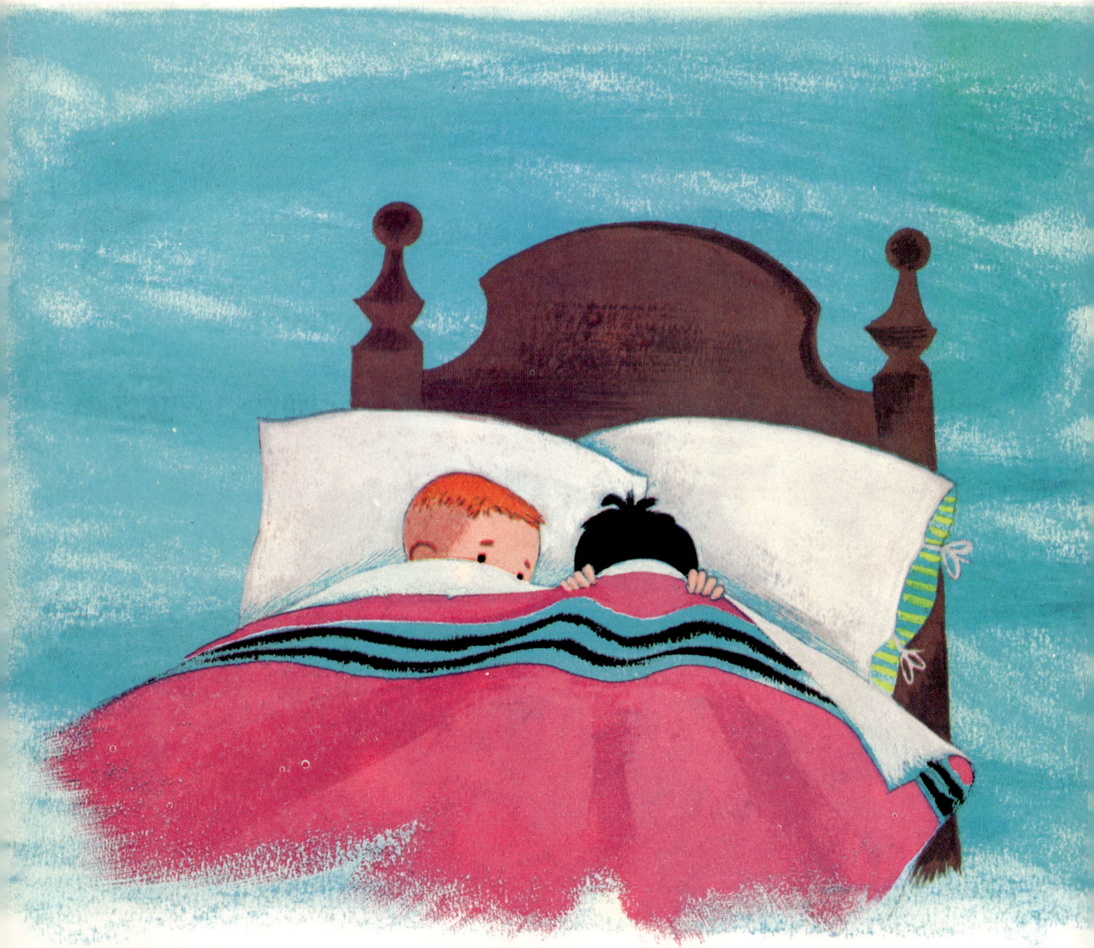

“Lie still,” said Mike.

“The man cannot see us. Do not be scared.”

The man saw Mike and Bill.

Mike peeked at him.

do

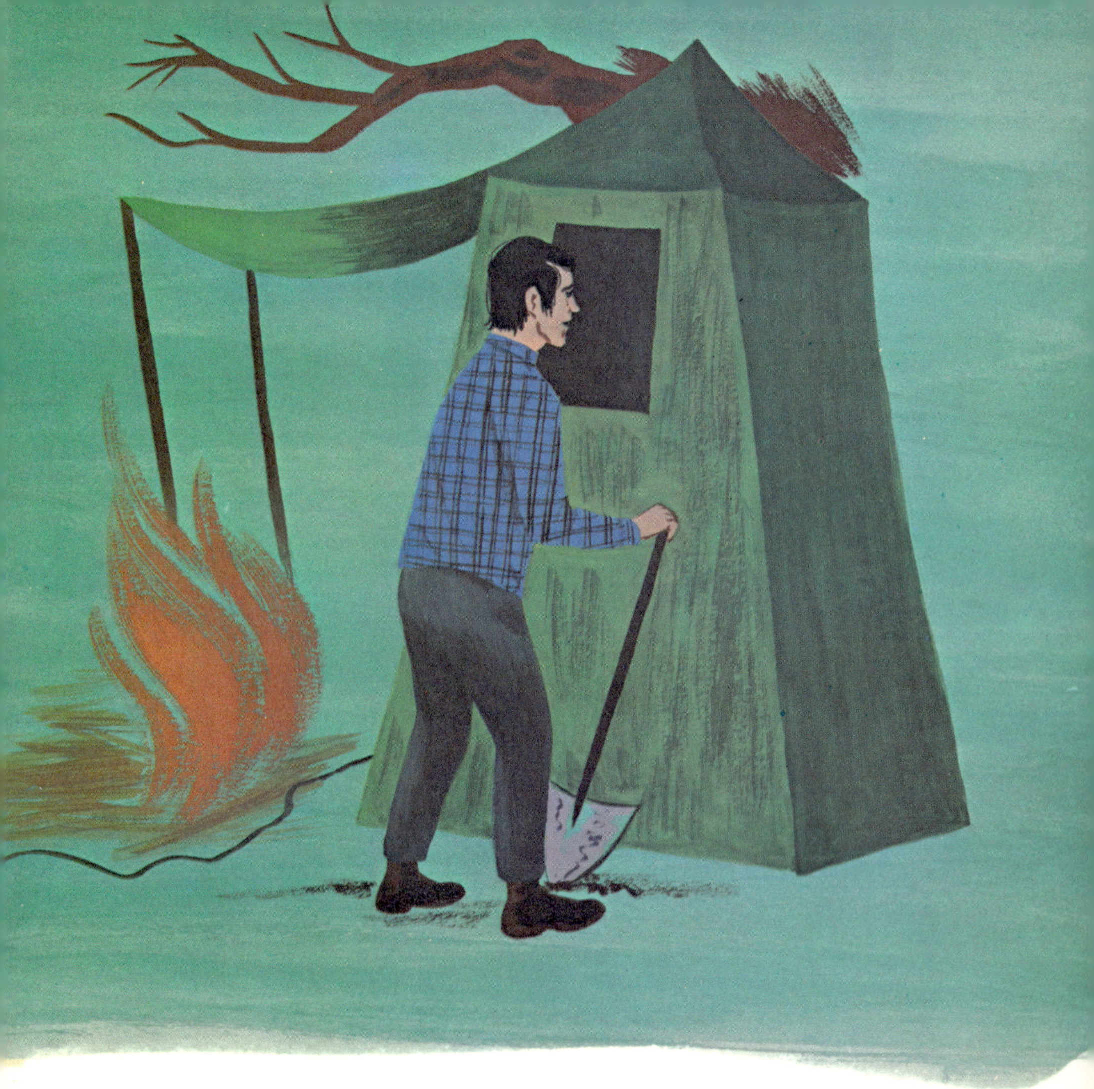

"Wake up, Mike," cried the man.

"The tent is on fire."

Mike and Bill ran from the tent. Bill saw the man first.

It was Farmer Tom.

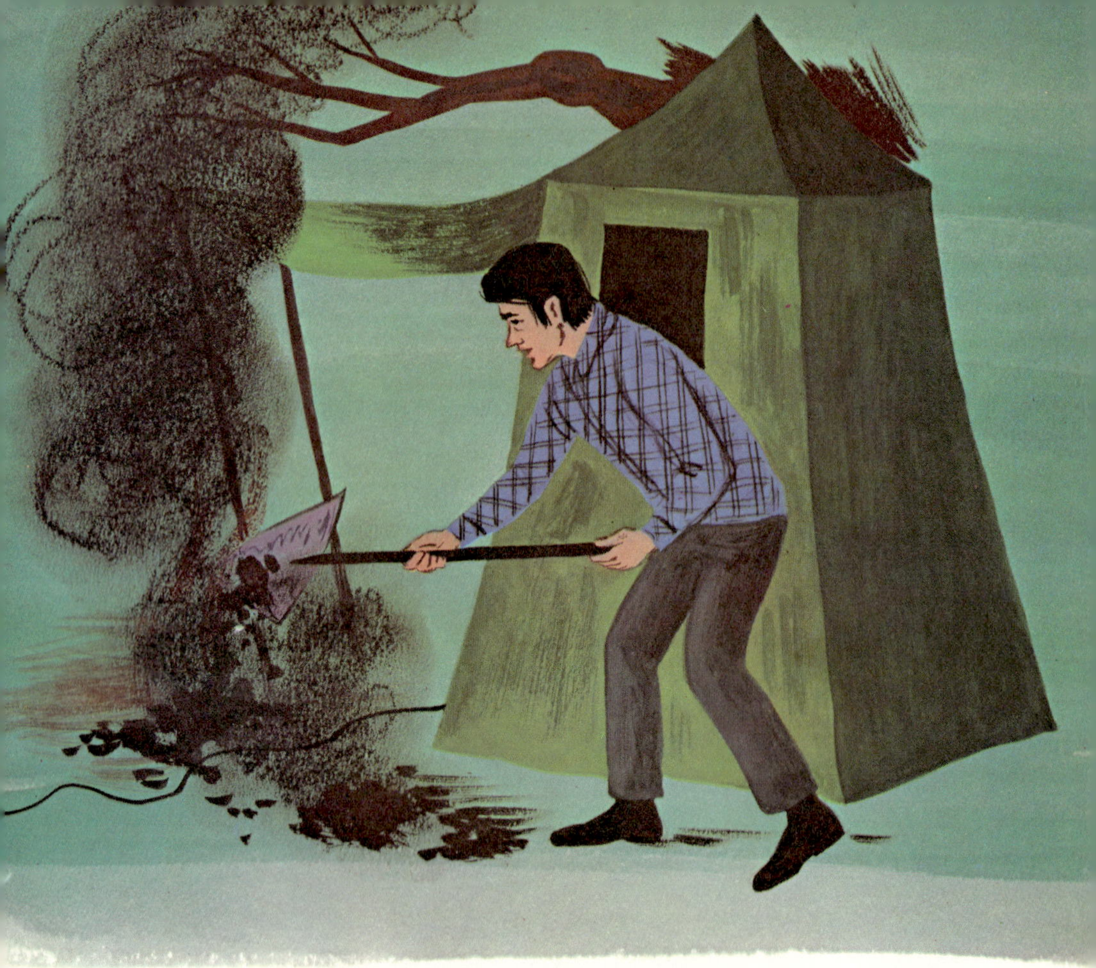

He had a spade.

He dug and tossed dirt on the fire.

"Farmer Tom is a fine man," said Bill.

"He came in time to stop the fire."

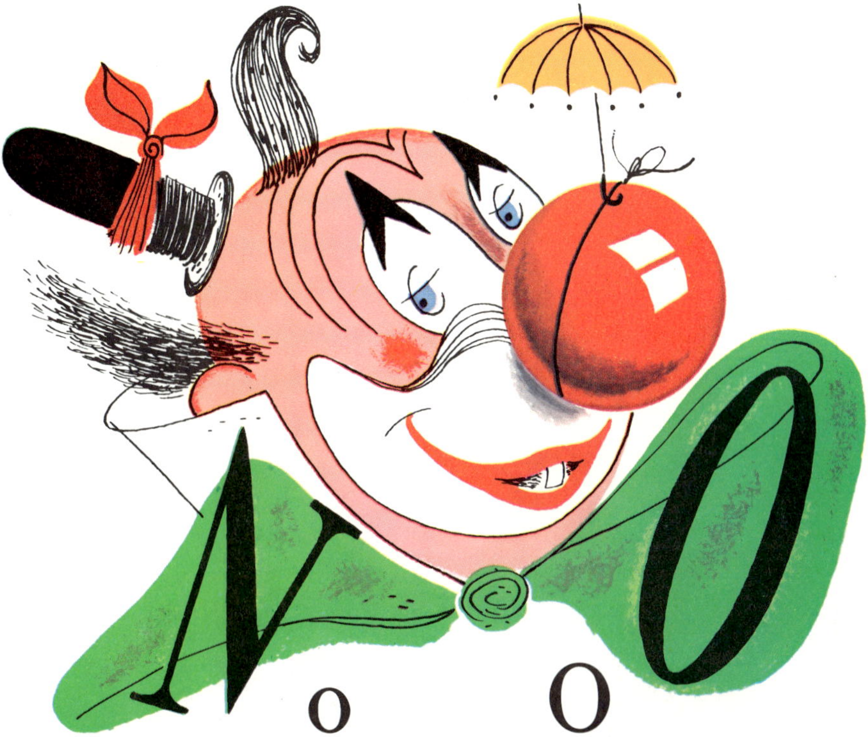

go no so

hole mole sole lone pole home
bone cone alone stone rode robe
smoke globe hope note poke stole
rose rope dose dome lope nose
tone drone

post most colt bolt host

holster poster old hold told

come some done

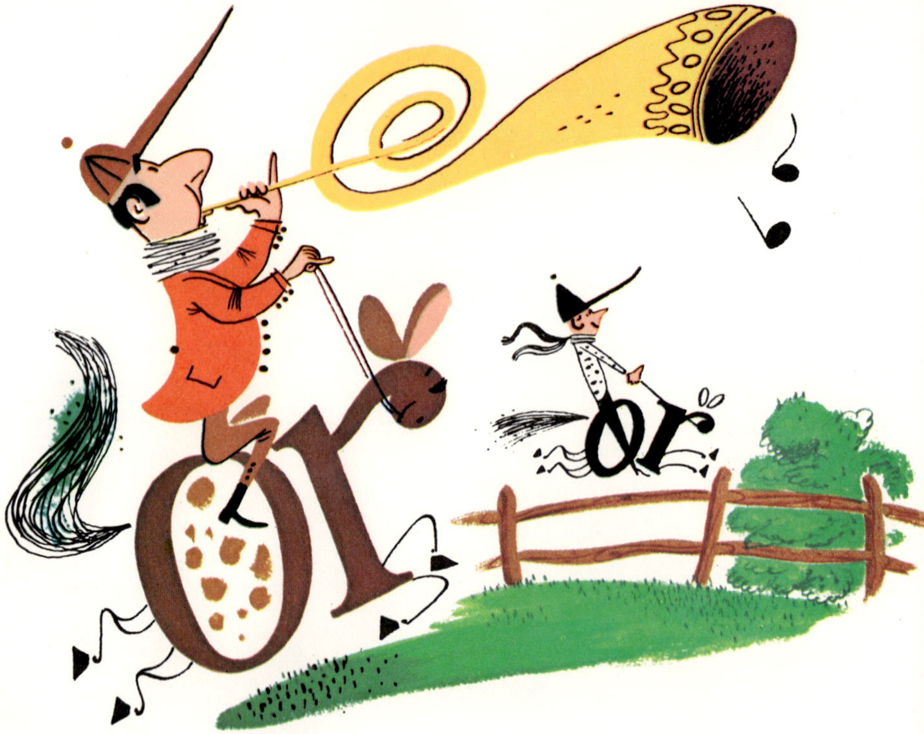

ore　　or

ore	more	core	wore
sore	bore	tore	before

or	nor	for	fork	corn
horn	born	torn	worn	cord
cork	lord	horse	acorn	corral

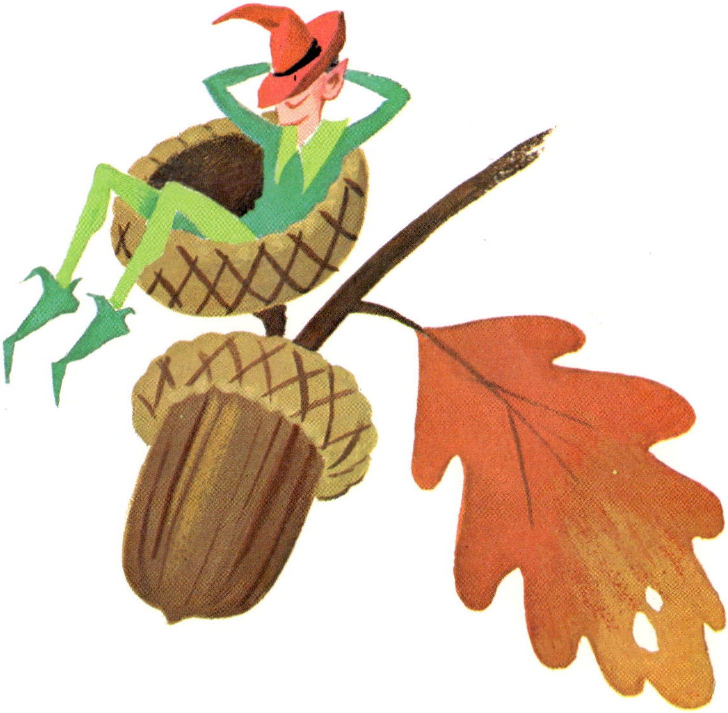

A little elf
Sat by himself
  Alone,
Alone in the lap
Of an acorn cap
  At home.

Adele H. Seronde

by

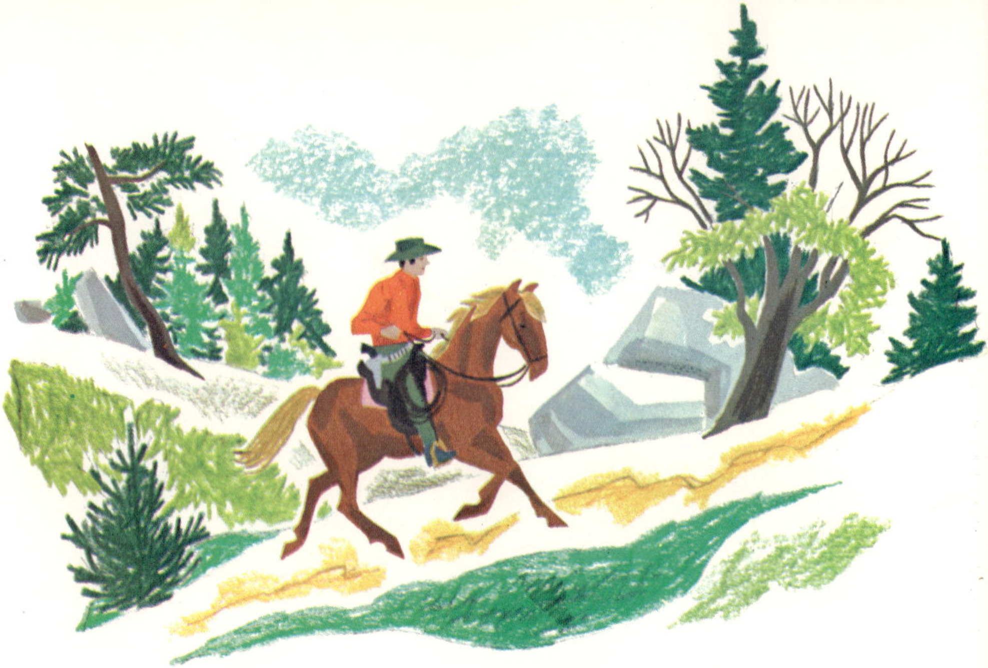

The Lost Cow

Carlos Calero rode his horse into the hills.

He went to find a lost cow.

Carlos wore a gun.

He had taken his braided rope from its nail near the corral. He had put the rope on his saddle.

He wanted to rope the lost cow and take her back home.

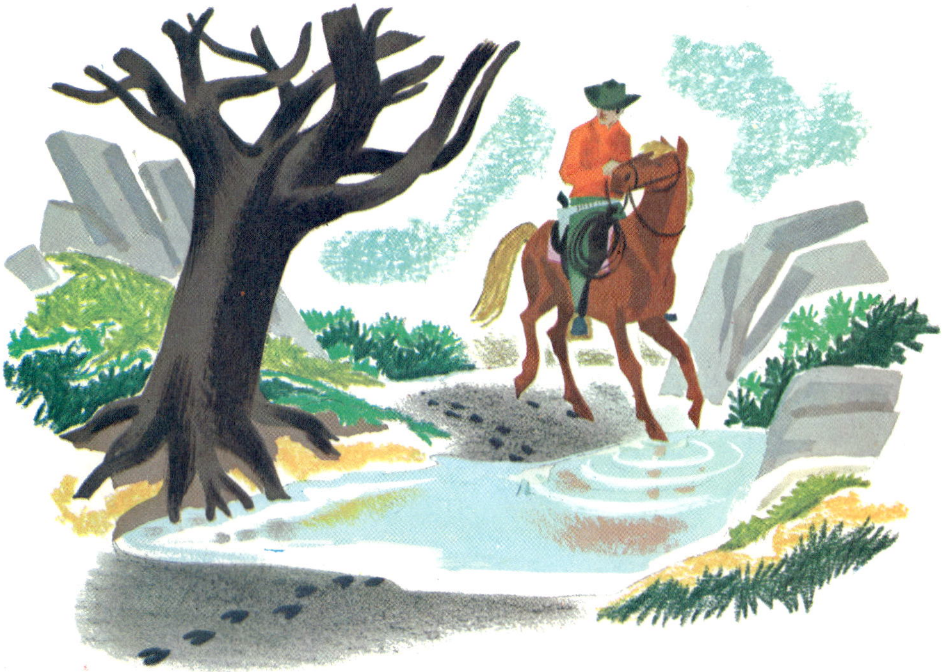

Carlos came to a water hole.

He saw some tracks his cow had made in the mud.

"I hope the lost cow is near," said Carlos. "I want to find her before dark."

Carlos saw more and more tracks in the sand and in the wet grass.

"Now I will find the cow," said Carlos. "Her tracks go here."

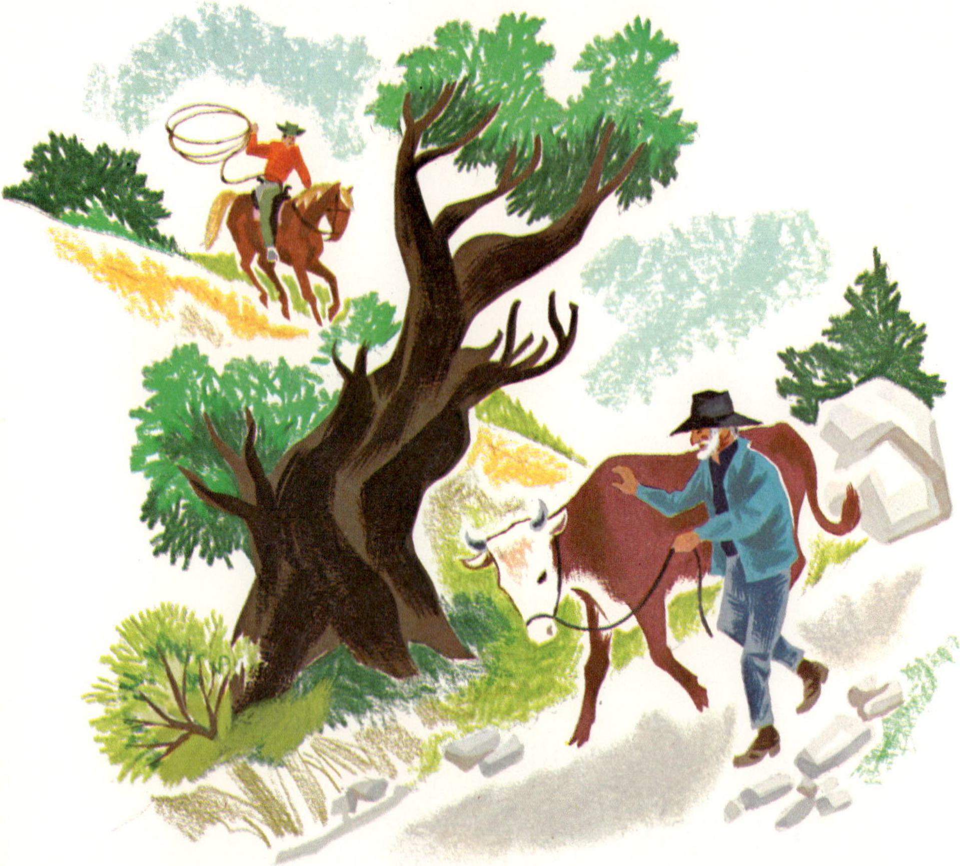

Carlos rode to the top of a big hill.

He saw a man and a cow.

"The man stole my cow," said Carlos. "I will take her from him."

Carlos started down the big hill.

He had his rope in his hand.

my

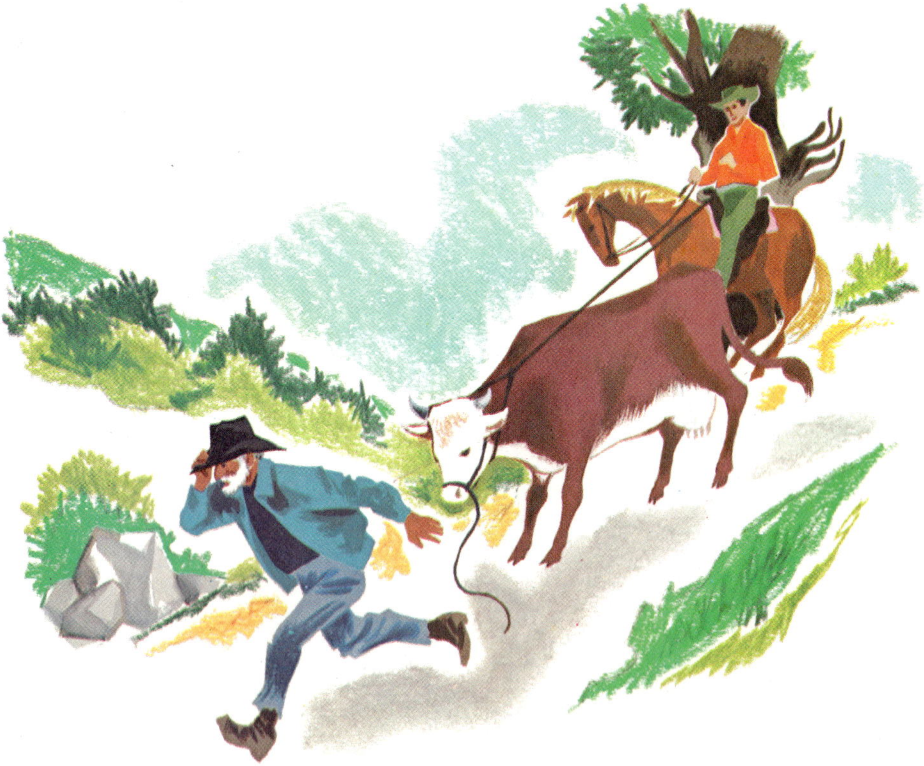

"Stop!" Carlos cried.

The man did not stop.

Carlos spun his rope in the air and made it sail at the man.

"I hope I can rope the man and the cow," he said.

Carlos got the cow in his rope.

"Now I can take the cow home," said Carlos. "The bad man will not get her."

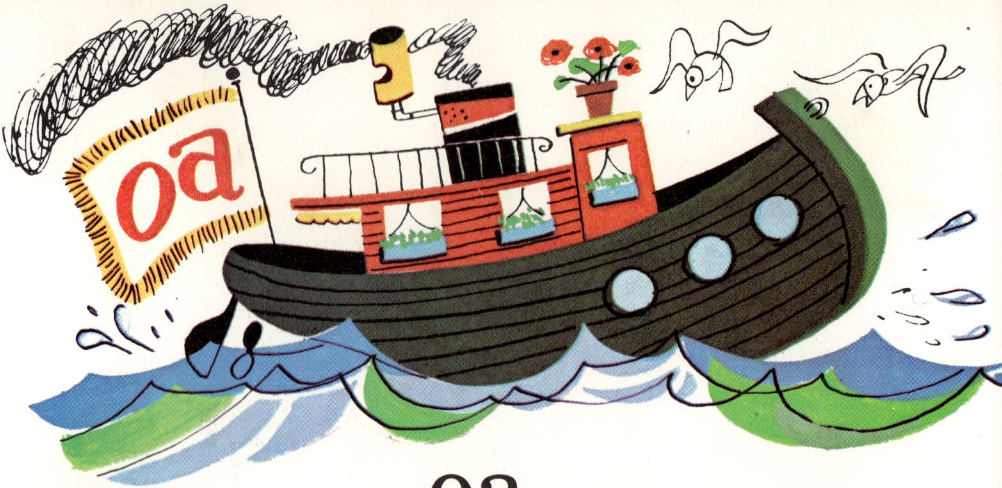

oa

oak oat boat coat goat soap
road toad soak foam roam loaf
coal goal moan groan cloak croak

oar roar soar board coarse hoarse

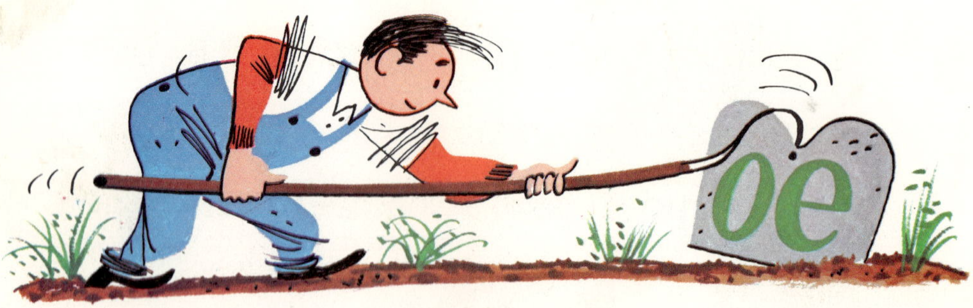

oe

toe foe hoe woe goes
does

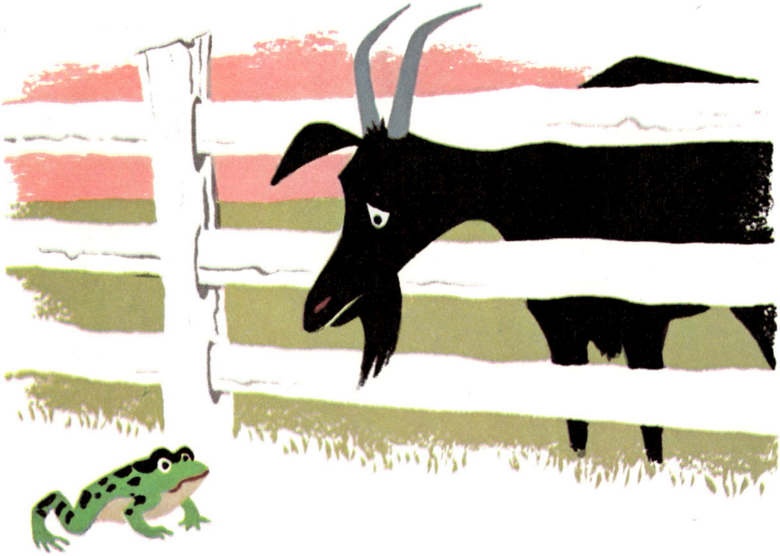

The Sad Goat

Once upon a time a goat sat near the side of a road. He was an old, fat goat.

The goat saw a green toad go down the road. "I want to hop like a toad," said the fat old goat. "I want to hop, hop, hop down the road."

once

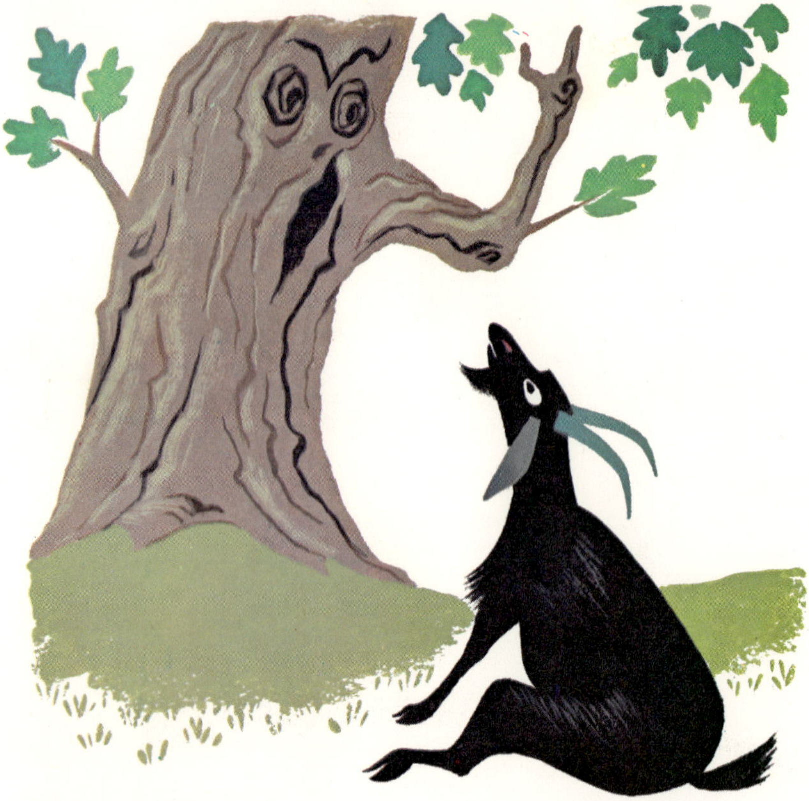

"A fat goat cannot hop," said the oak tree. "A frog can hop like a toad, but a fat goat cannot hop at all."

"I can hop if I want to," said the goat. "I will leap into the road now."

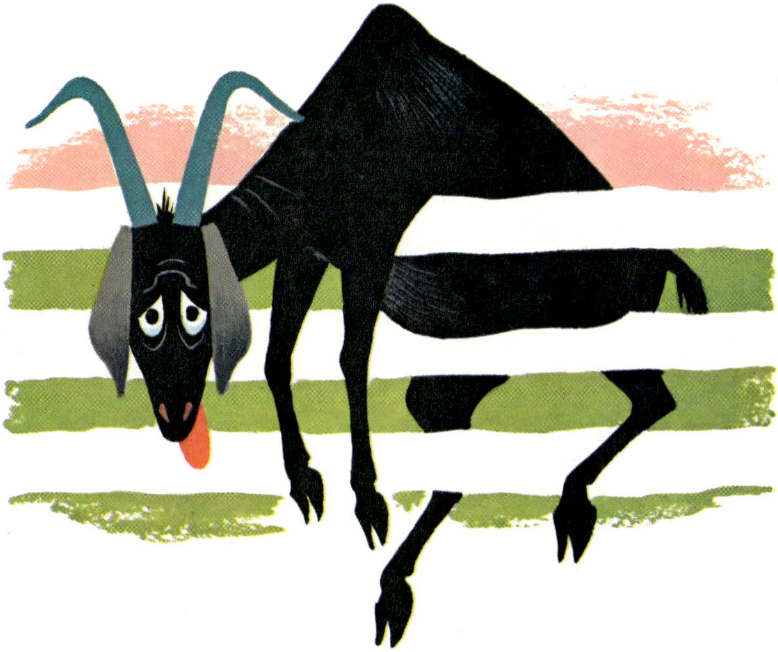

The old goat made a big leap for a fat goat. But he did not land on the road.

"Help me!" said the goat. "Help me get down from here! I cannot hop like a toad! I hop like a fat goat."

"The goat will not boast now," said the tall oak tree. "He will not boast how far he can leap."

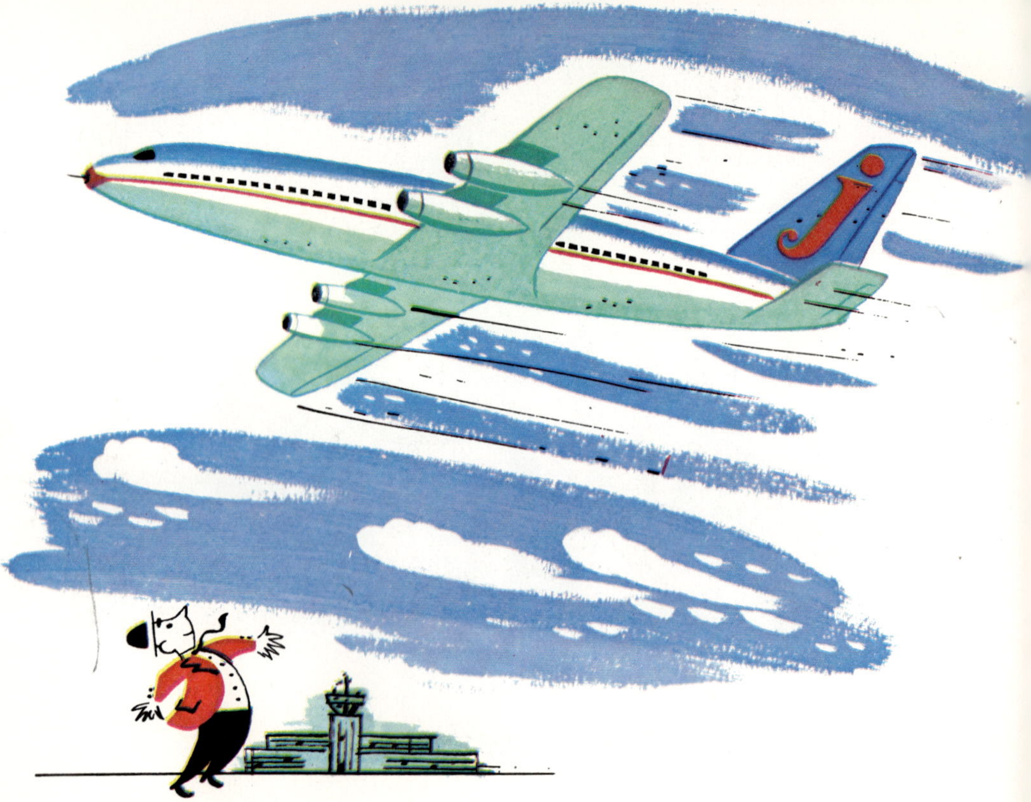

j J

jet	jig	jar	jag
job	Jeff	jog	jam
just	jug	James	jerk

jump	Jess	jaw	jot
Jack	Jim	Jones	joke
Jill	Jean	jab	junk
Jan	jeep	jail	Joan

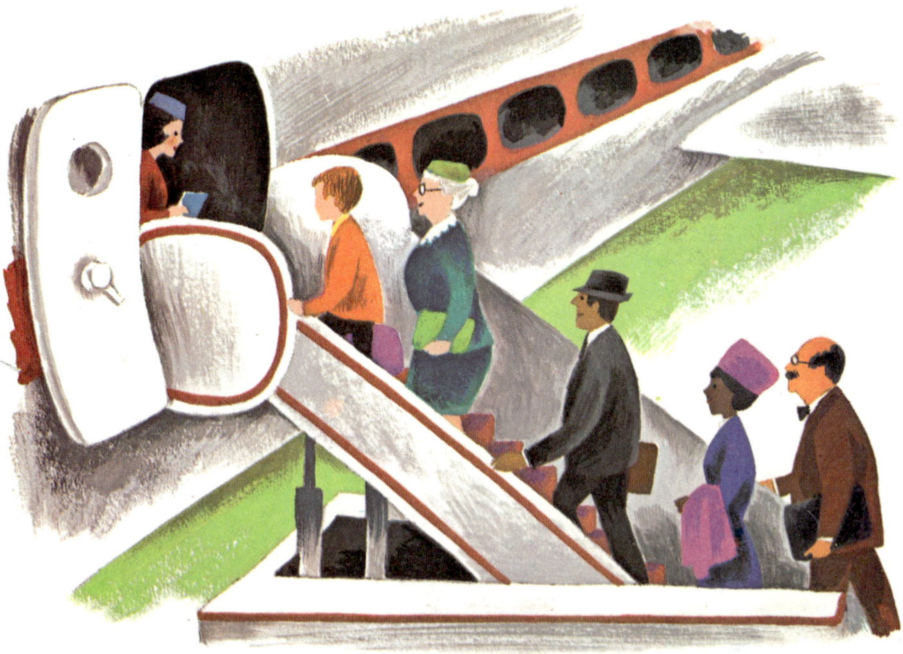

Ride in a Jet Plane

Jack went on a trip in a jet plane. It was his first plane ride. He went to see Jan. Jan's home was in West Falls.

A jet plane is big and it goes fast. It is as sleek as a bird. Jack had not seen a plane as big as the Star Fire.

The big plane sat still and Jack went up the steps.

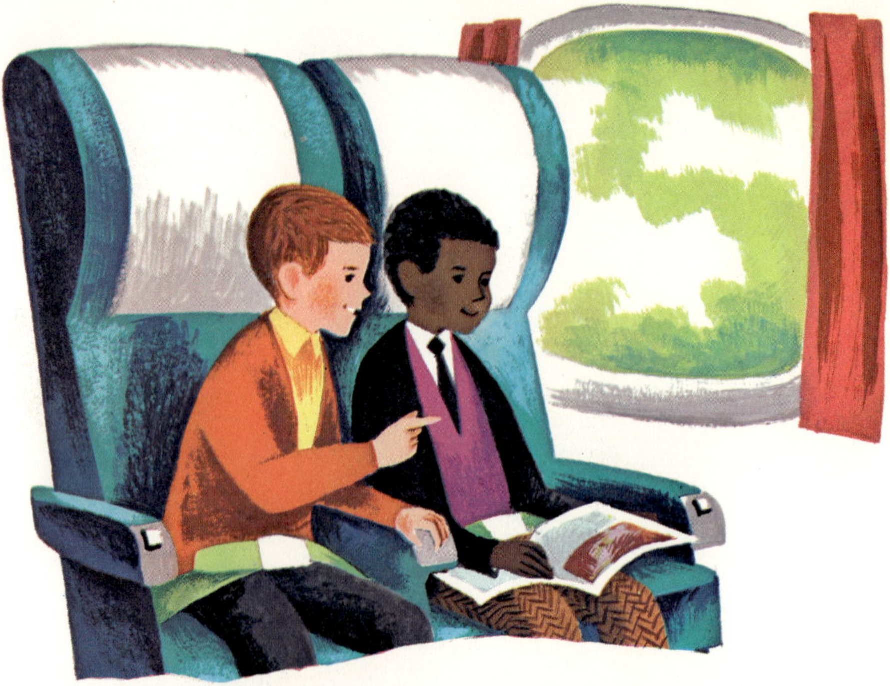

Jack sat beside James. James smiled at Jack. Jack smiled at James.

"We must lock the seat belts," said James.

Jack and James saw the pilot in the cockpit. His job was to pilot the Star Fire. The big plane started and went up, up, up.

"See how little the cars and trucks are," said Jack.

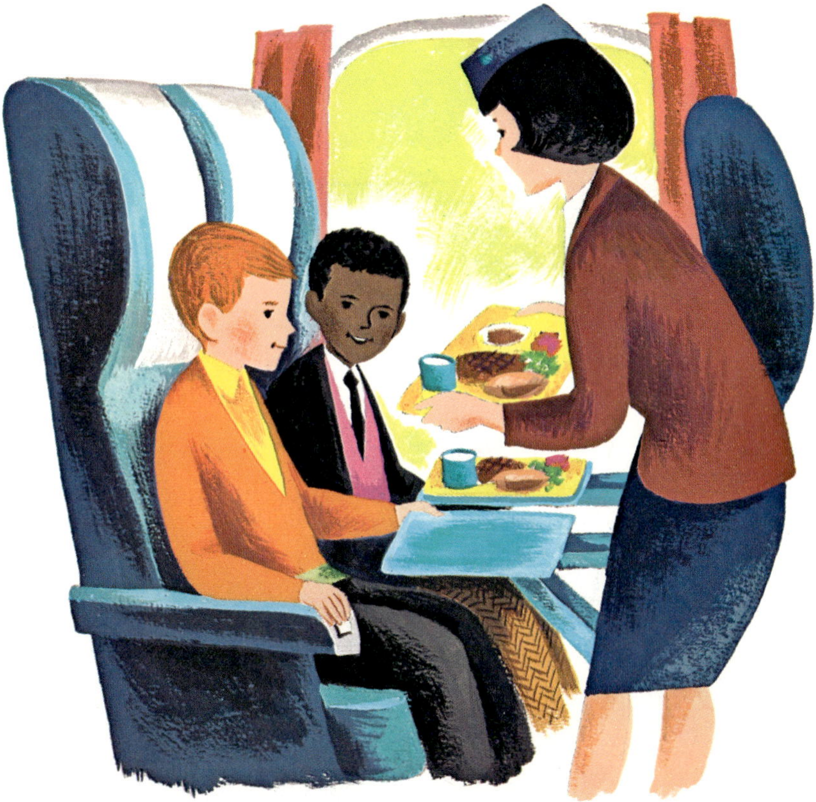

"Press the little button and the seat will go back or forward," said James.

"Here is dinner," said the hostess.

"Dinner on a jet is fun," said James.

"Just like home!" said Jack. "We can eat, read, or sleep if we want to."

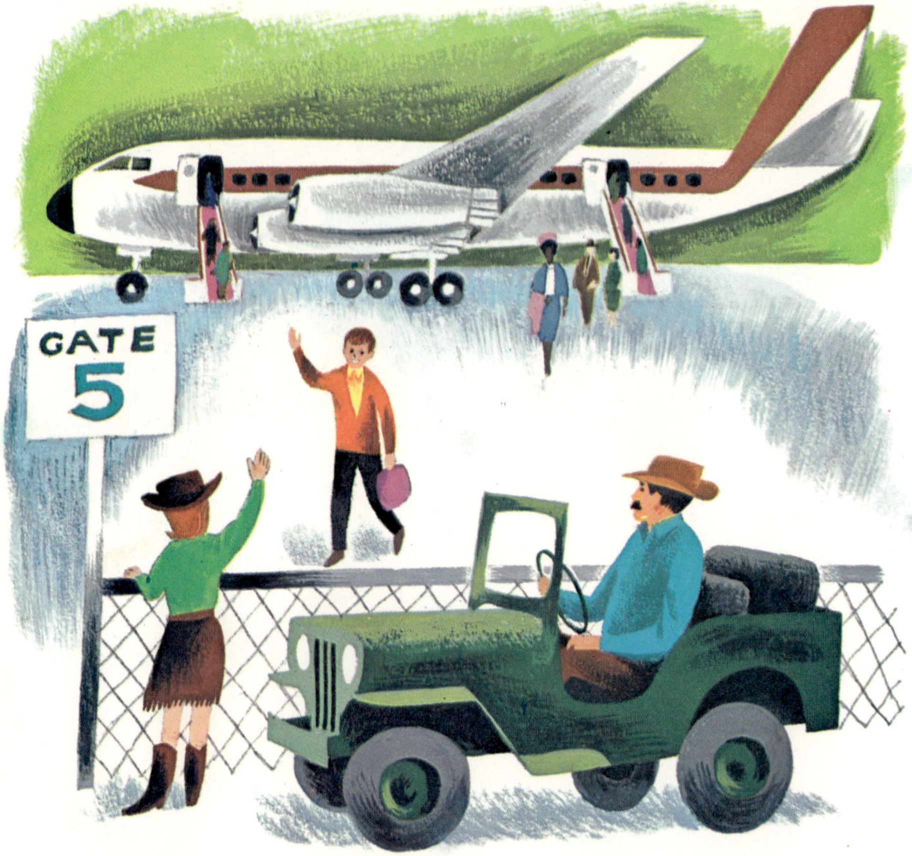

The Star Fire came to West Falls on time. Jack ran down the steps.

Jan came in a jeep to meet Jack and take him home.

"I had fun on the big jet plane," Jack told Jan.

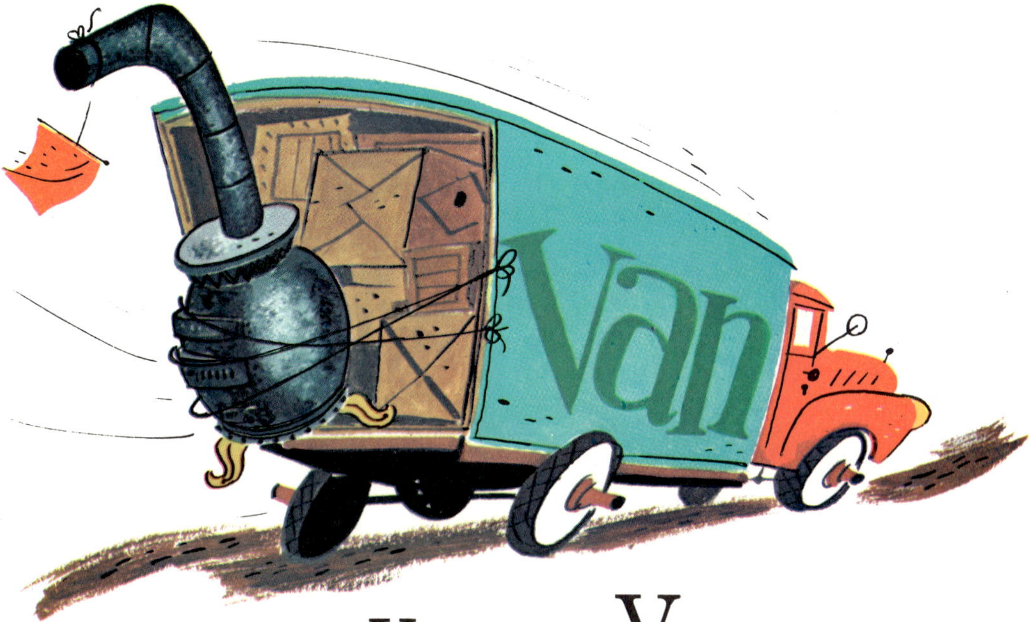

v V

van	stove	five	save
vent	alive	wave	over
vest	dive	wove	Rover
vile	gave	leave	diver
vote	pave	weave	vacant
volt	cave	cove	silver
vow	hive	eave	sliver

live	give	love	move
liver	have	glove	dove

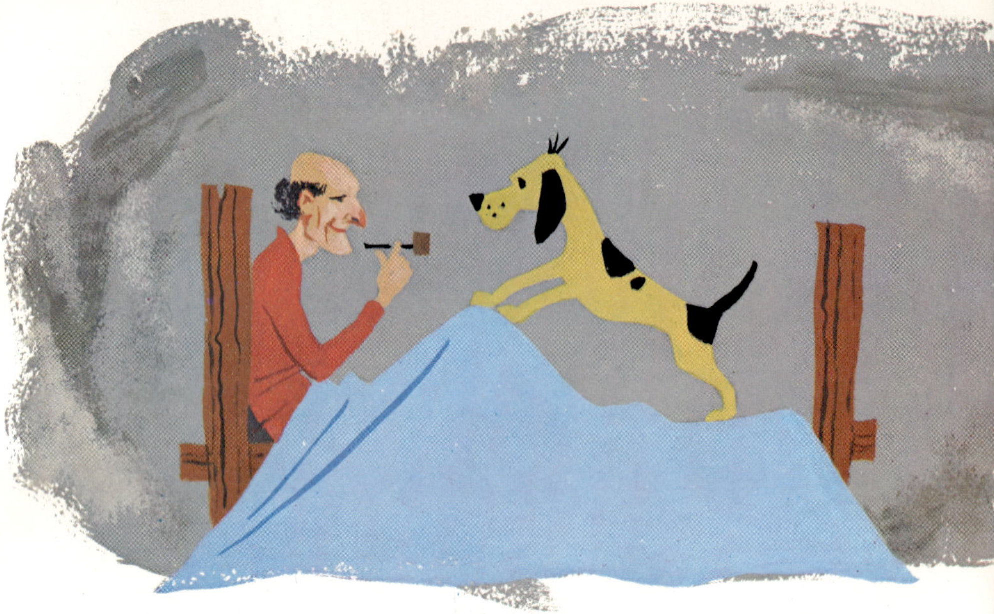

Van's Cave

Van is an old, old man. He lives in a cave near a lake. Van has a bed and a stove in the cave.

Van made the bed of old lumber. He made the stove of old bricks. He sleeps in the bed. Spot likes to sleep near the stove. His bed is just an old coat.

Spot likes to live in Van's cave. It is home for the old man and the dog.

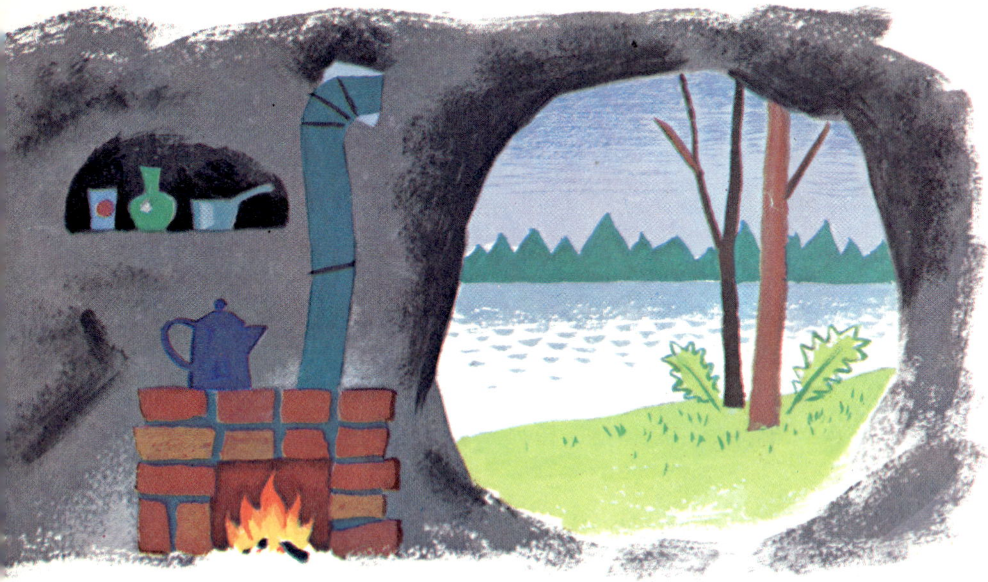

Once Van and Spot went to hunt ducks. Van saw a flock of ducks land on the lake. He fired and fired at the ducks.

"I hit five ducks," said Van. "Jump into the water, Spot, and get the ducks for me."

Spot jumped into the waves and swam to get the ducks.

"Fine dog," said Van. "We will eat the five ducks."

Van and Spot went back to the cave. Van made a fire.

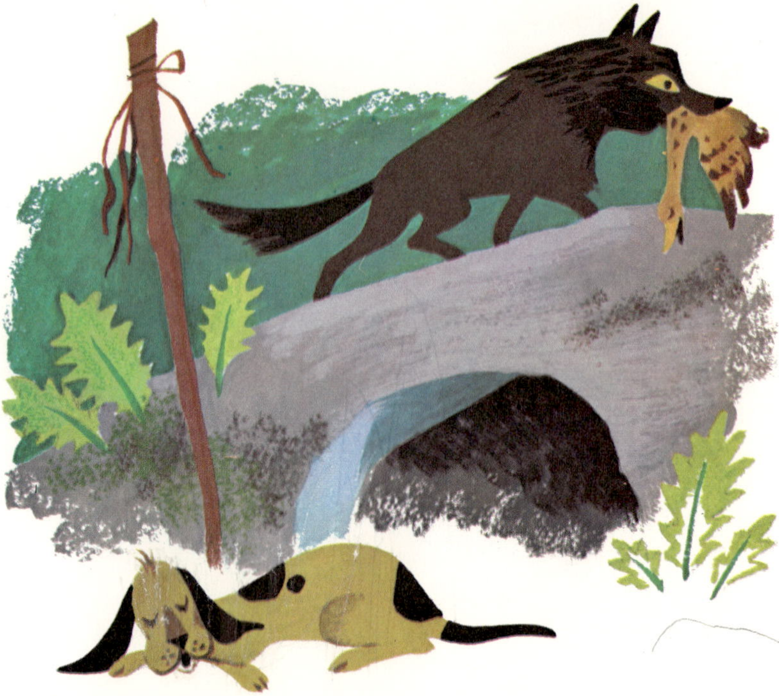

Spot must not leave the ducks.

He lies down near the cave.

"The fire is hot," said Van. "I will roast the ducks now."

Van did not see his five ducks. And Spot was fast asleep.

"Bad dog," said Van. "Now we must go and get more ducks."

Phoneme-grapheme Sequence in Books A – D

Book A

Sound	Page	Sound	Page	Sound	Page
short a	1	p	12	hard g	29
n	2	short i	15	hard c	32
r	3	s	18	h	36
d	5	short o	20	f	39
short u	7	t	22		
m	9	short e	25		

Book B

Sound	Page	Sound	Page	Sound	Page
ar	1	le	34	ai	58
er	5	k	37	long i, ie	64
ed	6	ck	39	ir	65
w	9	nk	41	long o	71
aw	19	signal e	44	ore, or	72
ow(cow)	24	a(care)	45	oa	78
l	26	long a	46	oe	78
ll	27	long e,ee	50	j	82
b	33	ea	54	v	87

Book C

Sound	Page	Sound	Page	Sound	Page
sh	1	-ing	33–38	dg,dge	89
ch,tch	5	-ed	44–47	-tion,-sion	97
th	8	er as er	52	oo(cook)	102
wh	14	ar as er	53	oo(food)	102
qu	17	ir,or,ur as er	54	ow(snow)	115
x	18	-y,-ay	64	ow(cow)	118
y	19	-ey	64	ou	119
z	20	soft c	75	long u	130
ng	26	soft g	88	ue,ui	130

Book D

Sound	Page	Sound	Page	Sound	Page
oi	1	kn	26	ea as long a	62
oy	1	silent b	36	ear	62
ew,eau	8	silent l	36	ie as long e	72
aw,au	14	silent g	48	ei as long e	72
ph as f	18	silent h	48	ei as long a	78
hard ch	18	silent gh	48	eigh as long a	78
ch as sh	18	gh as f	48	ey as long a	78
wr	26	ea as short e	62	ough	101

Acknowledgments

Illustrations: Ann Atene, Ruth and Allan Eitzen, Les Gray, Roland V. Shutts, Carol Wilde, and George Wilde.
Cover design: Phil Rath.

CONTENTS

Printed in the United States of America

ISBN-0-397-43537-1

82.5.775.6

BOOK B

BASIC READING

GLENN McCRACKEN
New Castle, Pennsylvania

CHARLES C. WALCUTT
Queens College, Flushing, New York

J. B. LIPPINCOTT COMPANY
PHILADELPHIA, NEW YORK